गोरक्ष संहिता

Goraksha Samhita

Also known as
Goraksha Paddhati

The Yogic Path of Guru Gorakshanatha

(English Translation Accompanied by Sanskrit
Text in Roman Transliteration)

Translated into English by
Swami Vishnuswaroop

Published by

Divine Yoga Institute

Kathmandu, Nepal

This book is dedicated to my Guru Swami Satyananda Saraswani,
Founder of Bihar School of Yoga,
Munger, India.

Contents

Gratitude

First of all I would like to express my heartfelt salutations to Adinatha (the Primordial Master) and my Guru Swami Satyananda Saraswati for their unwavering inspiration and guidance I have received for my work. I realize that my firm faith and belief in God and Guru is a motivational gift for me in completing this work. I could never have done it without their blessings.

I am always thankful to Ms. Bhawani Uprety for her untiring support she has provided me during my involvement in writing and translating various classical texts on yoga. My due thanks goes to her forever.

On the occasion of the Guru Purnima Day I wish that may God and Guru inspire us to tread the path of yoga in order to achieve the ultimate goal of human life!

- Swami Vishnuswaroop

Introduction

Gorakṣa Samhitā is composed by the great *Yogī Gorakṣanātha*. Renowned spiritual masters in the East have highly acknowledged and honored him as a *Siddha Yogī* for many centuries. His name is mentioned by *Svāmi Svātmārāma* in his classical text *Hatha Yoga Pradipikā* (Chapter One, Verses 4 and 5). He is also one of the Masters mentioned in the *Purānas* and yogic texts. He is well known as Guru *Gorakhanātha*, and a highly respected, revered and worshipped spiritual master in India and Nepal. The followers of the *Nātha* Tradition worship him as the incarnation of Lord *Śiva*, and say that the nine *Nāthas* and eighty-four *Siddhas* belong to *Adinātha*, Lord *Śiva*. So, he is also called *Śiva Gorakṣa*, the founder of the *Natha Siddha* tradition.

It is said that *Gorakṣanātha* was an Eighth Century *Siddha Yogī*. But some say that his physical presence occurred somewhere from the 8th to 11th century. According to the *Natha Siddha* tradition, Guru *Gorakhnātha* is an immortal sage and takes care of human beings and their welfare.

Gorkha, a historic district of Nepal, was named after *Gorakhanātha*, and its inhabitants were called Gorkhāli according to the legend. There is a cave of Guru *Gorakhnātha* which lies next to the famous *Gorakhakāli* Temple. Like Gorkha, the district of Gorakhapur in North Bihar of India, was also named after him. There is also a famous temple of *Gorakhanātha* in Gorakhapur.

It is said that *Hatha Yogī Mastsyendranāth* was the Guru of *Gorakṣanātha*. *Yogī Mastsyendranāth* received Yoga *Vidyā* (knowledge/wisdom) directly from the mouth of Lord *Śiva* through *Parvati*. It was Guru *Gorakṣanātha* who summarized the yogic subject matter in two hundred verses, which he had received from his Guru *Mastsyendranāth*, based on the teachings of *Śri Ādinātha* (Lord *Śiva*). This summarized text by *Gorakṣanātha* is called *Gorakṣa Samhitā* (compendium) which is also known as *Gorakṣa Paddhati: Yogic* Path of *Guru Gorakhanātha*.

Swami Vishnuswaroop

Gorakśa Samhitā highly emphasizes the purification of the body, *prāna* and the mind. It is believed that total purification of all impurities on both the physical and *prānic* levels is absolutely necessary in order to purify the mind. When these impurities are eliminated from the body and the energy blocks are removed, then the foundation for the awakening of the *Śakti* is prepared.

Therefore, *Guru Gorakhanātha* in *Gorakśa Samhitā* clearly outlines the various aspects of the *Hatha Yoga* practices e.g. *āsana, prānāyāma, mudrā, bandha* and *dhyāna*, etc., which serve as a solid foundation for the preparation and practice of *Raja Yoga*. Originally, the science of *Hatha Yoga* was discovered for the expansion and evolution of human consciousness, and for the accomplishment of the ultimate goal of human life, *mokśa* (liberation) through *samādhi* (the super conscious state).

According to *Gorakśa Samhitā*, the objective of *Hatha Yoga* is to create a harmonious balance between the physical body, *prāna* (the vital energy) and the mind. It is said that when the impulses generated by this harmonious balance stimulate the awakening of the *Kuṇḍalī Śakti*, only then is the evolution of consciousness or union between *Śiva* and *Śakti* possible. This accomplishment is the sole objective of the teaching of *Gorakśa Samhitā* by *Guru Gorakśanātha*.

It should be noted that the original Sanskrit Text is in Devanagari along with its Roman transliteration. All the Sanskrit words/phrases that appear in the English translation are given in the transliterated Roman alphabets.

It is hoped that this compilation will be helpful to all yoga lovers, yoga *sādhakas*, yoga teachers and yoga professionals to understand the traditional yoga, its objective and practice for the human welfare.

Publisher

Pūrva Śatakam

पूर्व शतकम्

Part One

Salutation to Guru

श्रीगुरुं परमानन्दं वन्दे स्वानन्दविग्रहम् ।

यस्य संनिध्यमात्रेण चिदानन्दायते तनुः ॥१॥

śrīgurum paramānandam vande svānandavigraham /

yasya sannidhyamātreṇa cidānandāyate tanuḥ //1//

I salute the teacher, who is in *paramānanda* (supreme bliss), and an embodiment of *svānanda* (self-bliss). Just by being near him, I find myself in a state of bliss. -1.1

नमस्कृत्य गुरुं भक्त्या गोरक्षो ज्ञानमुत्तमम् ।

अभीष्टं योगिनां ब्रूते परमानन्दकारकम् ॥२॥

namaskṛtya gurum bhaktyā gorakṣo jñānamuttamam /

abhīṣṭaṃ yogināṃ brūte paramānandakārakam //2//

Having expressed his devotion by saluting his Guru, *Gorakṣa* imparts the supreme knowledge, which is beneficial for all yogīs, and bestows ultimate bliss. -1.2

Objective of Gorakṣa Samhitā

गोरक्षसंहितां वक्ति योगिनां हितकाम्यया ।

ध्रुवं यस्यावबोधेन जायते परमं पदम् ॥३॥

gorakṣasaṃhitāṃ vakti yogināṃ hitakāmyayā /

dhruvaṃ yasyāvabodhena jāyate paramaṃ padam //3//

He will now expound the *Gorakṣa Samhitā* with his good wishes for the benefit of all yogīs. By understanding it, one will certainly attain *paraṃpada* (the supreme state). -1.3

एतद् विमुक्तिसोपानमेतत् कालस्य वञ्चनम् ।

यद् व्यावृत्तं मनो भोगादासक्तं परमात्मनि ॥४॥

etad vimuktisopānametat kālasya vañcanam /

yad vyāvṛttaṃ mano bhogādāsaktaṃ paramātmani //4//

This *Samhitā* is a ladder of liberation, and a way to deceive death. It turns the mind away from the attachment of *bhoga* (worldly pleasures) towards *Paramātma* (the Supreme Self). -1.4

Taking Refuge in Yoga

द्विजसेवितशाखस्य श्रुतिकल्पतरोः फलम् ।

शमनं भवतापस्य योगं भजत सत्तमाः ॥५॥

dvijasevitaśākhasya śrutikalpataroḥ phalam /

śamanaṃ bhavatāpasya yogaṃ bhajata sattamāḥ //5//

The most exceptional ones take refuge in yoga to relieve their worldly pains and sufferings. This branch of revelation (*śruti*) which is served by the *dvija* (literally, twice-born) yields the fruit of *kalpataru* (a heavenly tree that fulfills all one's wishes). -1.5

Six Limbs of Yoga

आसनं प्राणसंरोधः प्रत्याहारश्च धारणा ।

ध्यानं समाधिरेतानि योगाङ्गानि वदन्ति षट् ॥६॥

āsanaṃ prāṇasaṃrodhaḥ pratyāhāraśca dhāraṇā /

dhyānaṃ samādhiretāni yogāṅgāni vadanti ṣaṭ //6//

Āsana, control over *prāna, pratyahāra, dhārana, dhyāna* and *samādhi* are said to be the six limbs of yoga. -1.6

आसनानि च तावन्तो यावन्तो जीवजान्तवः ।

एतेषामखिलान् भेदान् विजानाति महेश्वरः ॥७॥

āsanāni ca tāvanto yāvanto jīvajāntavaḥ /

eteṣāmakhilān bhedān vijānāti maheśvaraḥ //7//

There are as many postures as there are sentient beings. *Maheśvara* (Lord *Śiva*) alone knows all their many forms. -1.7

Descriptions of Āsanas

चतुराशीतिलक्षाणामेकैकं समुदाहृतम् ।

ततः शिवेन पीठानां षोडेशानं शतं कृतम् ॥८॥

caturāśītilakṣāṇāmekaikaṃ samudāhṛtam /

tataḥ śivena pīṭhānāṃ ṣoḍeśānaṃ śataṃ kṛtam //8//

Of the eighty four hundred thousand āsanas, one hundred thousand have been mentioned. Thus Lord *Śiva* created eighty-four āsanas (*pithas*). -1.8

आसनेभ्यः समस्तेभ्यो द्वयमेतदुदाहृतम् ।

एकं सिद्धासनं प्रोक्तं द्वितीयं कमलासनम् ॥९॥

āsanebhyaḥ samastebhyo dvayametadudāhṛtam /

ekaṃ siddhāsanaṃ proktaṃ dvitīyaṃ kamalāsanam //9//

Among all the āsanas, two are mentioned specifically. The first is called *siddhāsana,* and the second is *kamalāsana* (i.e. *padmāsana*). -1.9

Siddhāsana

योनिस्थानकमङ्घ्रिमूलघटितं कृत्वा दृढं विन्यसेन्

मेढ्रे पादमथैकमेव हृदये कृत्वा हनुं सुस्थिरम् ।

स्थाणुः संयमितेन्द्रियो चलदृशा पश्येद् भ्रुवोरन्तरम्

ह्येतन्मोक्षकवाटभेदजनकं सिद्धासनं प्रोच्यते ॥१०॥

yonisthānakamaṅghrimūlaghaṭitaṃ kṛtvā dṛḍhaṃ vinyasen

meḍhre pādamathaikameva hṛdaye kṛtvā hanuṃ susthiram /

sthāṇuḥ saṃyamitendriyo caladṛśā paśyed bhruvorantaram

hyetanmokṣakavāṭabhedajanakaṃ siddhāsanaṃ procyate //10//

A yogī should firmly place his heel against *yonisthāna* (the perineum i.e. the base of urethra), while placing the other heel above the penis and pressing the chin against *hṛdaya* (the chest). With his senses restrained, the yogī should direct a steady gaze between the eyebrows. This is called *siddhāsana*, which breaks open the door to liberation. -1.10

Padmāsana

वामोरूपरि दक्षिणं चे चरणं संस्थाप्य वामं तथा

दक्षोरूपरि पश्चिमेनविधिना धृत्वा कराभ्यां दृढम् ।

अङ्गुष्ठौ हृदये निधाय चिबुकं नासाग्रमालोकयेद्

एतद् व्याधिविकारनाशनकरं पद्मासनं प्रोच्यते ॥११॥

vāmorūpari dakṣiṇam ce caraṇaṃ saṃsthāpya vāmaṃ tathā

dakṣorūpari paścimena vidhinā dhṛtvā karābhyāṃ dṛḍham /

aṅguṣṭhau hṛdaye nidhāya cibukaṃ nāsāgramālokayed

etad vyādhivikāranāśanakaraṃ padmāsanaṃ procyate //11//

One should place the right foot and leg on top of the left thigh and the left foot and leg on top of the right thigh. Then, crossing the hands behind the back, grasp the big toes properly. After placing the chin on the chest in the heart region, fix the gaze at the tip of the nose. This is called *padmāsana*, which destroys all types of diseases and health disorders. -1.11

Bodily Organs to Be Known

षट्चक्रं षोडशाधारं द्विलक्ष्यं व्योमपञ्चकम् ।

स्वदेहे ये न जानन्ति कथं सिद्ध्यन्ति योगिनः ॥१२॥

ṣaṭcakraṃ ṣoḍaśādhāraṃ dvilakṣyaṃ vyomapañcakam /

svadehe ye na jānanti kathaṃ siddhyanti yoginaḥ //12//

How can yogīs achieve perfection if they do not know the six *chakras* (energy centers), the sixteen supports of the body, the two objects of concentration and the five elements located within their own bodies? -1.12

एकस्तम्भं नवद्वारं गृहं पञ्चाधिदैवतम् ।

स्वदेहे ये न जानन्ति कथं सिद्ध्यन्ति योगिनः ॥१३॥

ekastambhaṃ navadvāraṃ gṛhaṃ pañcādhidaivatam /

svadehe ye na jānanti kathaṃ siddhyanti yoginaḥ //13//

How can yogīs be successful if they do not know that their own body is made from a single pillar, a home having nine doors and containing five *adhidevatā* (i.e. *ishtadevatā*, deities who fulfill one's desires)? -1.13

Description of Six Cakras

चतुर्दलं स्यादाधारः स्वाधिष्ठानं च षट्दलम् ।

नाभौ दशदलं पद्मं सूर्यसङ्ख्यदलं हृदि ॥१४॥

caturdalaṃ syādādhāraṃ svādhiṣṭhānaṃ ca ṣaṭdalam /

nābhau daśadalaṃ padmaṃ sūryasaṅkhyadalaṃ hṛdi //14//

The *ādhāra* (*mūladhāra*) *cakra* has four petals, and the *svādhiṣṭhāna cakra* has six. At the navel is a lotus with ten petals; at the heart, a lotus with twelve petals (*sūrya saṅkhya dalaṁ*, i.e. representing the twelve solar months). -1.14

कण्ठे स्यात् षोडशदलं भ्रूमध्ये द्विदलं तथा ।

सहस्रदलम् आख्यातं ब्रह्मरन्ध्रे महापथे ॥१५॥

kaṇṭhe syāt ṣoḍaśadalaṃ bhrūmadhye dvidalaṃ tathā /

sahasradalamākhyātaṃ brahmarandhre mahāpathe //15//

At the throat is a sixteen-petalled lotus; between the eyebrows, a lotus with two petals. At the *brahmarandhra* (literally, the hole or way to *Brahma*), which is also called *mahāpatha* (the supreme way), there is a lotus with a thousand petals. 1.15

आधारः प्रथमं चक्रं स्वाधिष्ठानं द्वितीयकम् ।

योनिस्थानं द्वयोर्मध्ये कामरूपं निगद्यते ॥१६॥

ādhāraṃ prathamaṃ cakraṃ svādhiṣṭhānaṃ dvitīyakam /

yonisthānaṃ dvayormadhye kāmarūpaṃ nigadyate //16//

The first energy center is *mūlādhāra*, and the second is *svādhiṣṭhāna*. Located between those two centers is the yoni (literally, source or origin), which is known as the seat of *kāma* (sensual desires). -1.16

आधाराख्यं गुदस्थानं पङ्कजं च चतुर्दलम् ।

तन्मध्ये प्रोच्यते योनिः कामाक्षा सिद्धवन्दिता ॥१७॥

ādhārākhyaṃ gudasthānaṃ paṅkajaṃ ca caturdalam /

tanmadhye procyate yoniḥ kāmākṣā siddhavanditā //17//

The lotus called *ādhārā* has four petals, and is located at the anus. It is said that in the middle of this lotus is the yoni *kāmākṣā*, which is greatly admired by the *siddhas*. – 1.17

The Supreme Light

योनिमध्ये महालिङ्गं पश्चिमाभिमुखस्थितम् ।

मस्तके मणिवद् बिम्बं यो जानाति स योगवित् ॥१८॥

yonimadhye mahāliṅgaṃ paścimābhimukhasthitam /

mastake maṇivad bimbaṃ yo jānāti sa yogavit //18//

In the middle of that yoni is a *mahāliṅga* (the great symbol of *Śiva*), which is facing backward. Its radiance is like a jewel on top of a head. One who knows it, knows Yoga. -1.18

तप्तचामीकराभासं तडिल्लेखेन विस्फुरत् ।

त्रिकोणं तत्पुरं वह्नरधो मेढ्रात्प्रतिष्ठितम् ॥१९॥

taptacāmīkarābhāsaṃ taḍillekheva visphurat /

trikoṇaṃ tatpuraṃ vahniradho medhrātpratiṣṭhitam //19//

The city of fire, which is in the shape of a triangle, is situated below the penis, and emanates flashes like lightning bolts, in the color of melted gold. -1.19

यत् समाधौ परं ज्योतिरनन्तं विश्वतोमुखम् ।

तस्मिन् दृष्टे महायोगे यातायातन्न विन्दते ॥२०॥

yat samādhau paraṃ jyotiranantaṃ viśvatomukham /

tasmin dṛṣṭe mahāyoge yātāyātanna vindate //20//

One who sees this Supreme Infinite Light, the form of the universe, in his *samādhi*, is the supreme yoga. After having seen that Great Light, he does not know his *yātāyataṁ* (literally, going and coming; i.e. he becomes liberated from the cycle of death and birth). -1.20

स्वशब्देन भवेत्प्राणः स्वाधिष्ठानं तदाश्रयः ।

स्वाधिष्ठानात्पदादस्मान्मेद्ध्रमेवाभिधीयते ॥२१॥

svaśabdena bhavetprāṇaḥ svādhiṣṭhānaṁ tadāśrayaḥ /

svādhiṣṭhānātpadādasmānmedhramevābhidhīyate //21//

The life force arises with the sound '*sva*', and its abode is the *svādhiṣṭhāna cakra*. This is thus called *medhra* (*liṅga*), as it takes refuge at *svādhiṣṭhāna*. -1.21

तन्तुना मणिवत्प्रोतो यत्र कन्दः सुषुम्णया ।

तन्नाभिमण्डलं चक्रं प्रोच्यते मणिपूरकम् ॥२२॥

tantunā maṇivatproto yatra kandaḥ suṣumṇayā /

tannābhimaṇḍalaṁ cakraṁ procyate maṇipūrakam //22//

The *chakra* located in the navel region is called *maṇipūra cakra*, where the *kanda* (bulbous root) is woven onto the *suṣumṇā* like a jewel on a thread. -1.22

द्वादशारे महाचक्रे पुण्यपापविवर्जिते ।

तावज् जीवो भ्रमत्य एव यावत् तत्त्वं न विन्दति ॥ २३॥

dvādaśāre mahācakre puṇyapāpavivarjite /

tāvajjīvo bhramatya eva yāvat tattvaṁ na vindati //23//

As long as *jīva* (the embodied self) wanders alone at the *mahācakra* (literally, great center) with twelve petals (the *manipura cakra*, located at the heart), which is free from *puṇya* (merit) and *pāpa* (demerit), the *jīva* does not know Reality. -1.23

Goraksha Samhita

Description of Ten Nādis

ऊर्ध्वं मेढ्रादधोनाभेः कन्दो योनिः खगाण्डवत् ।

तत्र नाड्यः समुत्पन्नाः सहस्राणां द्विसप्ततिः ॥२४॥

ūrdhvaṃ meḍhrādadhonābheḥ kando yoniḥ khagāṇḍavat /

tatra nāḍyaḥ samutpannāḥ sahasrāṇāṃ dvisaptatiḥ //24//

The *kanda yoni*, similar to a bird's egg, is located above the penis and below the navel. Seventy-two thousand *nādis* (subtle *prānic* channels) originate there. -1.24

तेषु नाडिसहस्त्रेषु द्विसप्ततिरुदाहृताः ।

प्रधानः प्राणवाहिन्यो भूयस्तासु दशस्मृताः ॥२५॥

teṣu nāḍisahasreṣu dvisaptatirudāhṛtāḥ /

pradhānāḥ prāṇavāhinyo bhūyastāsu daśasmṛtāḥ //25//

Among these thousands of *prānic* channels, seventy-two have been mentioned. Furthermore, among those seventy-two, ten are known as the most important carriers of *prāna*. -1.25

इडा च पिङ्गला चैव सुषुम्णा च तृतीयका ।

गान्धारी हस्तिजिह्वा च पूषा चैव यशस्विनी ॥२६॥

iḍā ca piṅgalā caiva suṣumṇā ca tṛtīyakā /

gāndhārī hastijihvā ca pūṣā caiva yaśasvinī //26//

Those channels called *iḍā* and *piṅgalā*, with *suṣumṇā* being the third one, *gāndhārī* and *hastijihvā*, *pūṣā* and *paśasvinī*. -1-26

अलम्बुषा कुहूश्चैव शङ्खिनी दशमी स्मृता ।

एतन्नाडिमयं चक्रं ज्ञातव्यं योगिभिः सदा ॥२७॥

alambuṣā kuhūścaiva śaṅkhinī daśamī smṛtā /

11

etannāḍimayaṃ cakraṃ jñātavyaṃ yogibhiḥ sadā //27//

The other channels are *alambuṣā* and *kuhūśa*, followed by *śaṅkhinī*, which is tenth. Yogīs should always have knowledge of each *cakra*, which is filled with these *prāṇic* channels. -1.27

Other Various Nādis

इडा वामे स्थिता भागे पिङ्गला दक्षिणे स्थिता ।

सुषुम्णा मध्यदेशे तु गान्धारी वामचक्षुषि ॥२८॥

iḍā vāme sthitā bhāge piṅgalā dakṣiṇe sthitā /

suṣumṇā madhyadeśe tu gāndhārī vāmacakṣuṣi //28//

Iḍā is situated on the left side and *piṅgalā* is on the right, while *suṣumṇā* is in the middle, while the *gāndhārī* is in the left eye. -1.28

दक्षिणे हस्तिजिह्वा च पूषा कर्णे च दक्षिणे ।

यशस्विनी वामकर्णे ह्यानने चाप्यलम्बुषा ॥२९॥

dakṣiṇe hastijihvā ca pūṣā karṇe ca dakṣiṇe /

yaśasvinī vāmakarṇe hyānane cāpyalambuṣā //29//

Hastijihvā is on the right and *pūṣā* is in the right ear, while *yaśasvinī* is in the left ear and *alambuṣā* is located in the mouth. -1.29

कुहूश्च लिङ्गदेशे तु मूलस्थाने च शङ्खिनी ।

एवं द्वारं समाश्रित्य तिष्ठन्ति दशनाडयः ॥३०॥

kuhūśca liṅgadeśe tu mūlasthāne ca śaṅkhinī /
evaṃ dvāraṃ samāśritya tiṣṭhanti daśanāḍayaḥ //29//

Kuhū is located in the region of the *liṅga* and the *śaṅkhinī* is located in the area of the anus. Thus the ten subtle *prāṇic* channels are supported by, and situated at, the portals of the body. -1.30

इडापिङ्गलासुषुम्णाः प्राणमार्गे समाश्रिताः ।

सततं प्राणवाहिन्यः सोमसूर्याग्निदेवताः ।।३१।।

iḍāpiṅgalāsuṣumṇāḥ prāṇamārge samāśritāḥ /

satataṃ prāṇavāhinyaḥ somasūryāgnidevatāḥ //31//

Iḍā, piṅgalā and *suṣumṇā* are associated with, and depend on, the path of *prāṇa* (i.e. life force). They are constant carriers of *prāṇa*, and their respective *devatās* (deities) are *soma* (the moon), *sūrya* (the sun) and *agni* (fire). -1.31

The Ten Vāyus

प्राणोऽपानः समानश्चोदानोव्यानौ च वायवः ।

नागः कूर्मोथ कृकलो देवदत्तो धनञ्जयः ।। ३२।।

prāṇo'pānaḥ samānaścodānovyānau ca vāyavaḥ /

nāgaḥ kūrmo'tha kṛkalo devadatto dhanañjayaḥ //32//

Prāṇa, apāna, samāna, udāna, vyāna, nāga, kūrma, kṛkara, devadatta and *dhanañjaya* are the ten *prāṇas* (vital life forces) in the body. 1.32

हृदि प्राणो वसेन्नित्यंअपानो गुदमण्डले ।

समानो नाभिदेशे तु उदानः कण्ठमध्यगः ।।३३।।

hṛdi prāṇo vasennityam apāno gudamaṇḍale /

samāno nābhideśe tu udānaḥ kaṇṭhamadhyagaḥ //33//

Prāṇa always dwells in the heart, *apāna* is in the region of the anus, *samāna* is in the navel region, and *udāna* is in the middle of the throat. -1.33

व्यानो व्यापी शरीरेषु प्रद्धानाः पञ्च वयवः ।

प्राणाद्याः पञ्चविख्याता नागाद्याः पन्च वयवः ।।३४।।

vyāno vyāpī śarīreṣu pradhānāḥ pañca vāyavaḥ /
prāṇādyāḥ pañcavikhyātā nāgādyāḥ pañca vāyavaḥ //34//

Vyāna pervades the whole body. These five *prāṇas* (life forces) are of great renown. Starting with *nāga*, below are the five other (sub) *prāṇas*. -1.34

उद्गारे नाग आख्यातः कूर्म उन्मीलने स्मृतः ।
कृकरः क्षुतकृज् ज्ञेयो देवदत्तो विजृम्भणे ।।३५।।

udgāre nāga ākhyātaḥ kūrma unmīlane smṛtaḥ /
kṛkaraḥ kṣutakṛjjñeyo devadatto vijṛmbhaṇe //35//

It is known that *nāgā* performs belching and *kūrma* blinking of the eyes, *kṛkara* causes hunger and thirst, and *devadatta* yawning and hiccupping. -1.35

न जहाति मृतं चापि सर्वव्यापि धनञ्जयः ।
एते सर्वासु नाडीषु भ्रमन्ते जीवरूपिणः ।।३६।।

na jahāti mṛtaṃ cāpi sarvavyāpi dhanañjayaḥ /
ete sarvāsu nāḍīṣu bhramante jīvarūpiṇaḥ //36//

Dhanañjaya pervades the whole body, and does not depart from it even after death. Therefore, *jīvarūpiṇa* (the embodied Self or Soul in the form of *jīva*) pervades all of these subtle life force channels. -1.36

आक्षिप्तो भुजदण्डेन यथोच्चलति कन्दुकः ।
प्राणापानसमाक्षिप्तस्तथा जीवो न तिष्ठति ।।३७।।

ākṣipto bhujadaṇḍena yathoccalati kandukaḥ /
prāṇāpānasamākṣiptastathā jīvo na tiṣṭhati //37//

As a ball struck with a stick goes up (and comes down), so the *jīva* (the embodied Self), when struck by *prāṇa* and *apāna*, does not remain still. -1.37

Need of Prāṇāpāna Practice

प्राणापानवशो जीवो ह्य् अधश् चोर्ध्वं च धावति ।

वामदक्षिणमार्गेण चञ्चलत्वान्न दृश्यते ॥३८॥

prāṇāpānavaśo jīvo hyadhaścordhvaṃ ca dhāvati /

vāmadakṣiṇamārgeṇa cañcalatvānna dṛśyate //38//

Being under the control of *prāṇa* and *apāna*, the *jīva* (embodied Self), traverses up and down through the left and right (*prānic*) pathways. Due to its restlessness, it does not perceive its own true form (the nature of the Self). -1.38

रज्जुबद्धो यथा श्येनो गतोऽप्याकृष्यते पुनः ।

गुणबद्धस्तथा जीवः प्राणापानेन कृष्यते ॥३९॥

rajjubaddho yathā śyeno gato'pyākṛṣyate punaḥ /

guṇabaddhastathā jīvaḥ prāṇāpānena kṛṣyate //39//

Like a hawk tied down with a string that can fly away, only to be pulled back again, so the *jīva*, bound by the *guṇas* (i.e. the qualities or modes of nature), is subject to the pull of *prāṇa* and *apāna*. -1.39

अपानः कर्षति प्राणः प्राणोपानं च कर्षति ।

ऊर्ध्वाधः संस्थितावेतौ संयोजयति योगवित् ॥४०॥

apānaḥ karṣati prāṇaṃ prāṇo'pānaṃ ca karṣati /

ūrdhvādhaḥ saṃsthitāvetau saṃyojayati yogavit //40//

The *apāna* draws the *prāṇā*, and the *prāṇā* draws the *apāna*. One who unites these two *prānas*, which are situated above and below (the navel area), is the knower of yoga. -1.40

Haṃsa Mantra and Ajapā Gāyatri

हकारेण बहिर्याति सकारेण विशेत्पुनः ।

हंसहंसेत्यमुं मन्त्रं जीवो जपति सर्वदा ॥४१॥

hakāreṇa bahiryāti sakāreṇa viśetpunaḥ /

haṃsahaṃsetyamuṃ mantraṃ jīvo japati sarvadā //41//

With the sound '*ha*', the *jīva*, in the form of *prāna*, goes out; with the sound '*sa*', it comes back in again. So the *jīva* is always repeating the mantra '*haṃsa, haṃsa*'. -1.41

षट्शतानि त्वहोरात्रे सहस्राण्येकविंशतिः ।

एतत्सङ्ख्यान्वितं मन्त्रं जीवो जपति सर्वदा ॥४२॥

ṣaṭsatāni tvahorātre sahasrāṇyekaviṃśatiḥ /

etatsaṅkhyānvitaṃ mantraṃ jīvo japati sarvadā //42//

In fact, the *jīva* continually recites this mantra 21,600 times in each diurnal cycle. -1.42

अजपा नाम गायत्री योगिनां मोक्षदायिनी ।

अस्याः सङ्कल्पमात्रेण सर्वपापैः प्रमुच्यते ॥४३॥

ajapā nāma gāyatrī yogināṃ mokṣadāyinī /

asyāḥ saṅkalpamātreṇa sarvapāpaiḥ pramucyate //43//

The *Gāyatrī* named *Ajapā* bestows liberation upon yogīs, and merely through its power of *saṅkalpa* (resolve or vow), one is released from all sins. -1.43

Note: *Saṅkalpa* means a definite intention, will or vow for doing something. Say a determination/resolution to do something.

अनया सदृशी विद्या अनया सदृशो जपः ।

अनया सदृशं ज्ञानं न भूतं न भविष्यति ।।४४।।

anayā sadṛśī vidyā anayā sadṛśo japaḥ /

anayā sadṛśaṃ jñānaṃ na bhūtaṃ na bhaviṣyati //44//

There is no *vidyā* (wisdom) similar to the *Gāyatrī* named *Ajapā*, there is no *japa* (recitation) similar to it, there is no *jñāna* (knowledge) similar to it, nor was there in the past, nor will there be in the future. -1.44

कुन्दलिन्याः समुद्भूता गायत्री प्राणधारिणी ।

प्राणविद्या महाविद्या यस्तां वेत्ति स योगवित् ।।४५।।

kuṇḍalinyāḥ samudbhūtā gāyatrī prāṇadhāriṇī /

prāṇavidyā mahāvidyā yastāṃ vetti sa yogavit //45//

One who knows this life-supporting *Gāyatrī* (i.e. *Ajapā*), born out of *kuṇḍalinī*, which is *prāṇavidyā* (knowledge) and *mahāvidyā* (supreme wisdom) of *prāṇa* (the life force), is the knower of yoga. -1.45

Awakening of Kuṇḍalī Śakti

कन्दोर्ध्वे कुण्डली शक्तिरष्टधा कुण्डलाकृति ।

ब्रह्मद्वारमुखं नित्यं मुखेनाच्छाद्य तिष्ठति ।। ४६।।

kandordhve kuṇḍalī śaktiraṣṭadhā kuṇḍalākṛti /

brahmadvāramukhaṃ nityaṃ mukhenācchādya tiṣṭhati //46//

The *kuṇḍalī śakti* (power), folded into eight coils, always resides above the *kanda* (bulbous root), closing the opening of the *brahmadvāra* (door of *Brahma*) with its face. -1.46

येन द्वारेण गन्तव्यं ब्रह्मागारमनामयम् ।
मुखेनाच्छाद्य तद्द्वारं प्रसुप्ता परमेश्वरी ॥४७॥

yena dvāreṇa gantavyaṃ brahmāgāramanāmayam /

mukhenācchādya taddvāraṃ prasuptā parameśvarī //47//

The way to *brahmāgāra* (the abode of *Brahma*), which is *anāmaya* (literally, free from any fault and disease), is through this door. But *Parameśvarī* (the Supreme Goddess) is asleep there, covering that door with her face. -1.47

प्रबुद्धा वह्नियोगेन मनसा मारुता सह ।
सूचीव गुणमादाय व्रजत्यूर्ध्वं सुषुम्णया ॥४८॥

prabuddhā buddhiyogena manasā mārutā saha /

sūcīva guṇamādāya vrajatyūrdhvaṃ suṣumṇayā //48//

When *kuṇḍalī* is awakened by intelligence, the mind and *maruta* (*prāṇa*) blend together, and she moves upwards through *suṣumṇā* (the middle pathway) like a needle drawing a thread. -1.48

प्रस्फुरद्भुजगाकारा पद्मतन्तुनिभा शुभा ।
प्रबुद्धा वह्नियोगेन व्रजत्यूर्ध्वं सुषुम्णया ॥४९॥

prasuptabhujagākārā padmatantunibhā śubhā /

prabuddhā vahniyogena vrajatyūrdhvaṃ suṣumṇayā //49//

When awakened by the yogic fire, she raises upwards through the *suṣumṇa* (middle path) in the form of a serpent, bursting up like an auspicious filament of a lotus. -1.49

उद्घाटयेत् कपातं तु यथा कुञ्चिकया हठात् ।
कुण्डलिन्या तथा योगी मोक्षद्वारं प्रभेदयेत् ॥५०॥

udghāṭayet kapāṭaṃ tu yathā kuñcikayā haṭhāt /

kuṇḍalinyā tathā yogī mokṣadvāram prabhedayet //50//

Just as one forcibly unlocks a door with a key, so the yogī should break open the door to liberation by means of the *kuṇḍalinī*. -1.50

Śakticālini Mudrā

कृत्वा सम्पुटितौ करौ दृढतरं बद्ध्वा तु पद्मासनं
गाढं वक्षसि सन्निधाय चिबुकं ध्यानं च तच्चेतसि ।
वारम्वारमपानमूर्ध्वमनिलं प्रोच्चारयेत्पूरितं
मुञ्चन्प्राणमुपैति बोधमतुलं शक्तिप्रभावादतः ॥५१॥

kṛtvā sampuṭitau karau dṛḍhataraṃ baddhvā tu padmāsanaṃ

gāḍhaṃ vakṣasi sannidhāya cibukaṃ dhyānaṃ ca taccetasi /

vāramvāramapānamūrdhvamanilaṃ proccārayetpūritaṃ

muñcunprāṇamupaiti bodhamatulaṃ śaktiprabhāvādataḥ //51//

After cupping the hands firmly and assuming the lotus posture while placing the chin tightly against the chest, one should practice meditation focusing his mind on *Tat* (*Brahma* in the Light Form), and after he has filled the chest with *prāna*, should repeatedly expel the *apāna vāyu*. Upon releasing the *prāna*, he acquires *bodhamatula* (incomparable knowledge) through the force of the awakening of *Śakti*. -1.51

Daily Routine of a Yogī

अङ्गानां मर्दनं कृत्व श्रमसञ्जातवारिणा ।
कट्वम्ललवणत्यागी क्षीरभोजनमाचरेत् ॥५२॥

aṅgānāṃ mardanaṃ kṛtva śramasañjātavāriṇā /

kaṭvamlalavaṇatyāgī kṣīrabhojanamācaret //52//

One should rub his limbs with the sweat caused by one's labors. One should consume milk and abstain from bitter, sour, and salty foods. -1.52

ब्रह्मचारी मिताहारी त्यागी योगपरायणः ।
अब्दाद्ऊर्ध्वं भवेत्सिद्धो नात्र कार्या विचारणा ॥५३॥

brahmacārī mitāhārī tyāgī yogaparāyaṇaḥ /

abdādūrdhvam bhavetsiddho nātra kāryā vicāraṇā //53//

One who is dedicated to the practice of yoga should be a *brahmacārī* (celibate) and a *tyāgī* (renouncer), and should be a *mitāhārī* (one who takes moderate diet). One will then achieve perfection after one year. There should be no doubt about it. -1.53

सुस्निग्धं मधुराहारं चतुर्थांशविवर्जितम् ।
भुज्यते स्वरसं प्रीत्यै मिताहारी स उच्यते ॥५४॥

susnigdham madhurāhāram caturthāṃśavivarjitam /

bhujyate svarasam prītyai mitāhārī sa ucyate //54//

One who is called a *mitāhārī* (literally, a moderate eater) eats food that is smooth, oil-rich, sweet and natural in taste after offering it to his God, and leaves one-fourth of his stomach empty. -1.54

कन्दोर्ध्वं कुण्डलीनी शक्ति शुभमोक्षप्रदायिनी ।
बन्धनाय च मूढानां यस्तां वेत्ति स योगवित् ॥५५॥

kandordhvam kuṇḍalīnī śakti śubhamokṣapradāyinī /

bandhanāya ca mūḍhānām yastām vetti sa yogavit //55//

Kuṇḍalīnī śakti, situated above the *kanda* (bulbous root), is the bestower of auspicious liberation for yogīs, but causes bondage for fools. One who realizes this is a knower of yoga. -1.55

Description of Mudrās

महामुद्रां नमोमुद्रां उड्डियानं जलन्धरम् ।

मूलबन्धनं च यो वेत्ति स योगी मुक्तिभाजनः ॥५६॥

mahāmudrāṃ nabhomudrāṃ uḍḍiyānaṃ jalandharam /

mūlabandhannīca yo vetti sa yogī muktibhājanaḥ //56//

A yogī who is familiar with the *mahāmudrā, nabhomudrā, uḍḍiyāna bandha, jalandhara bandha* and *mūlabandha* practices is worthy of liberation. -1.56

Mahāmudrā

वक्षोन्यस्तहनुः प्रपीड्य सुचिरं योनिं च वामाङ्घ्रिणा

हस्ताभ्यामवधारयेत् प्रसरितं पादं तथा दक्षिणम् ।

आपूर्य श्वसनेन कुक्षियुगलं बद्ध्वा शनैरेचयेत्

एषा व्याधिविनाशिनी सुमहती मुद्रा नृणां कत्यते ॥५७॥

vakṣonyastahanuḥ prapīḍya suciraṃ yoniṃ ca vāmāṅghriṇā

hastābhyāmavadhārayet prasaritaṃ pādaṃ tathā dakṣiṇam /

āpūrya śvasanena kukṣiyugalaṃ baddhvā śanaiḥ recayet

eṣā vyādhivināśinī sumahatī mudrā nṛṇāṃ kathyate //57//

Placing the chin on the chest, constantly pressing the left heel against the *yoni* (the perineum), and holding the extended right foot with the hands, the yogī should, after inhaling and holding the air fully inside the chest, exhale it slowly. It is said that this is an extremely great mudra, the destroyer of all human diseases. -1.57

चन्द्राङ्गेन समभ्यस्य सूर्याङ्गेनाभ्यसेत्पुनः ।

यावत्तुल्या भवेत्सङ्ख्या ततो मुद्रां विसर्जयेत् ॥५८॥

candrāṅgena samabhyasya sūryāṅgenābhyasetpunaḥ /

yāvattulyā bhavetsaṅkhyā tato mudrāṃ visarjayet //58//

After practicing the *mahāmudrā* first with *candrāṅga* (the lunar side/part, i.e. the left nostril), one should practice it with *sūryāṅga* (the solar side/part, i.e. the right nostril). One should stop this *mudrā* after practicing an equal number of rounds with both *aṅgas*. -1.58

Results of Mahāmudrā

नहि पथ्यमपथ्यं वा रसाः सर्वेऽपि नीरसाः ।

अपि मुक्तं विषं घोरं पीयूषमिव जीर्यते ॥५९॥

nahi pathyamapathyaṃ vā rasāḥ sarve'pi nīrasāḥ /

api bhuktaṃ viṣaṃ ghoraṃ pīyūṣamiva jīryate //59//

There is no wholesome or unwholesome food (for an expert yogī), and all tastes indeed are tasteless. Even eating a horrible poison is digested like *pīyūṣa* (nectar). -1.59

क्षयकुष्ठगुदावर्तगुल्माजीर्णपुरोगमाः ।

तस्य दोषाः क्षयं यान्ति महामुद्रां तु योऽभ्यसेत् ॥६०॥

kṣayakuṣṭhagudāvartagulmājīrṇapurogamāḥ /

rogāstasya kṣayaṃ yānti mahāmudrāṃ tu yobhyaset //60//

In addition, for one who practices the *māhamudrā*, diseases like leprosy, constipation, enlargement of the spleen, indigestion, etc. are destroyed. -1.60

कथितेयं महामुद्रा महासिद्धिकरा नृणाम् ।

गोपनीया प्रयत्नेन न देया यस्य कस्यचित् ॥६१॥

kathiteyaṃ mahāmudrā mahāsiddhikari nṛṇām /

gopanīyā prayatnena na deyā yasya kasyacit //61//

It is said that this *mahā mudrā* is the bestower of human perfections. With due effort, one should try to keep it secret. It should not be given to everyone. -1.61

Goraksha Samhita

Khecari Mudrā

कपालकुहरे जिह्वा प्रविष्टा विपरीतगा ।

भ्रुवोरन्तर्गता दृष्टिर् मुद्रा भवति खेचरी ॥६२॥

kapālakuhare jihvā praviṣṭā viparītagā /

bhruvorantargatā dṛṣṭirmudrā bhavati khecarī //62//

One should turn the tongue backward into the skull cavity, and fix the gaze between the two eyebrows. This is (the practice of) *khecarī mudrā.* -1.62

Results of Khecari Mudrā

न रोगान्मरणं तस्य न निद्रा न क्षुधा तृषा ।

न मूर्च्छा तु भवेत्तस्य यो मुद्रां वेत्ति खेचरीम् ॥६३॥

na rogānmaraṇaṃ tasya na nidrā na kṣudhā tṛṣā /

na mūrcchā tu bhavettasya yo mudrāṃ vetti khecarīm //63//

For one who knows *khecarī mudrā*, there is no disease, death, tiredness, sleep, hunger, thirst or fainting. - 1.63

पीड्यते न च शिकेन लिप्यते न च कर्मणा ।

बाध्यते न स केनापि यो मुद्रां वेत्ति खेचरीम् ॥६४॥

pīḍyate na ca śokena lipyate na ca karmaṇā /

bādhyate na sa kenāpi yo mudrāṃ vetti khecarīm //64//

One who knows *khecarī mudrā* is not affected by diseases or grief, nor tainted by his karma (actions). One cannot be obstructed by anything. -1.64

चित्तं चलति नो यस्माज्जिह्वा चरति खेचरी ।

तेनेयं खेचरी सिद्धा सर्वसिद्धैर्नमस्कृता ॥६५॥

cittaṃ calati no yasmājjihvā carati khecarī /

teneyaṃ khecarī siddhā sarvasiddhairnamaskṛtā //65//

As the tongue goes into *khecari* (i.e. into the cavity of the skull, or literally, moving in the region of sky), *citta* (the mind) does not move. Consequently, the perfected practice of *khecarī mudrā* is saluted by all the *siddhas*. -1.65

बिन्दुमूल शरीरणां शिरास्तत्र प्रतिष्ठिताः ।

भावयन्ति शरीराणमापादतलमस्तकम् ।।६६।।

bindumūlaṃ śarīraṇāṃ śirāstatra pratiṣṭhitāḥ /

bhāvayanti śarīrāṇamāpādatalamastakam //66//

Bindu (semen) is the foundation of all bodies in which the veins [in the physical body] and the *nādis* (in the *prāṇic* body) are established. They compose all bodies from the head to the feet. -1.66

खेचर्या मुद्रितं येन विवरं लम्बिकोर्ध्वतः ।

न तस्य क्षरते बिन्दुः कामिन्यालिङ्गितस्य च ।।६७।।

khecaryā mudritaṃ yena vivaraṃ lambikordhvataḥ /

na tasya kṣarate binduḥ kāminyāliṅgitasya ca //67//

For one who has sealed the cavity of the skull through the *khecarī mudrā*, semen is not ejaculated, even if he is embraced by an amorous woman. -1.67

यावद् बिन्दुः स्थितो देहे तावन्मृतोर्भयं कुतः ।

यावद् बद्धा नभोमुद्रा तावद् बिन्दुर्न गच्छति ।।६८।।

yāvad binduḥ sthito dehe tāvanmṛtorbhayaṃ kutaḥ /

yāvad baddhā nabhomudrā tāvad bindurna gacchati //68//

As long as the *bindu* remains in the body, how can there be fear of death? As long as *nabhomudrā* (meaning *khecarī mudrā*) is maintained, the *bindu* does not go out (of the body). -1.68

Making the Bindu Stable in Its Place

चलितोऽपि यदा बिन्दुः सम्प्राप्तश् च हुताशनम् ।

व्रजत्यूर्ध्वं हृतः शक्त्या निरुद्धो योनिमुद्रया ।।६९।।

calito'pi yadā binduḥ samprāptaśca hutāśanam /

vrajatyūrdhvaṃ hṛtaḥ śaktyā niruddho yonimudrayā //69//

Even if the semen has fallen into the *hutāśana* (literally, it means sacrifice eater or fire, i.e. located in the navel region), it should be taken upward again and controlled by the *Śakti* (power) of the yoni *mudrā*. -1.69

स पुनर्द्विविधो बिन्दुः पण्डुरो लोहितस्तथा ।

पाण्डुरः शुक्रमित्याहुर्लोहिताख्यो महाराजः ।।७०।।

sa punardvividho binduh paṇḍuro lohitastathā /

pāṇḍuraḥ śukramityāhurlohitākhyo mahārajaḥ //70//

In addition, *bindu* is of two kinds: yellowish white and red. It is said that the color of *śukra* (the semen) is yellowish white, and the great *raja* (ovarian fluid) is red. -1.70

सिन्दूरद्रवसङ्काशं नाभिस्थाने स्थितं रजः ।

शशिस्थाने स्थितो बिन्दुस्तयोरैक्यं सुदुर्लभम् ।।७१।।

sindūradravasankāśaṃ nābhisthāne sthitaṃ rajaḥ /

śaśisthāne sthito bindustayoraikyaṃ sudurlabham //71//

The *raja* is located in the navel area and resembles oil mixed with the color vermilion. The *bindu* is located at the place of the moon (i.e. at the palate). It is quite rare to unite them. -1.71

Supreme State: Unity of Bindu and Raja

बिन्दुः शिवो रजः शक्तिर्बिन्दुम् इन्दू रजो रविः ।

अनयोः सङ्गमादेव प्राप्यते परमं पदम् ॥७२॥

binduḥ śivo rajaḥ śaktiscandro bindū rajo raviḥ /

anayoḥ saṅgamādeva prāpyate paramaṃ padam //72//

Bindu is *Śiva* and *raja* is *Śakti. Bindu* is the moon and *raja* is the sun. One can accomplish *parama pada* (the Supreme State) through the union of these two. -1.72

वायुना शक्तिचारेण प्रेरितं तु यदा रजः ।

याति बिन्दोः सहैकत्वं भवेद्दिव्यं वपुस्ततः ॥७३॥

vāyunā śakticāreṇa preritam tu yadā rajaḥ /

yāti bindoḥ sahaikatvaṃ bhaveddivyaṃ vapustataḥ //73//

When the activating power of *vāyu* (*prāna*) stimulates *raja*, it unites with the *bindu*. Then, the body becomes divine. -1.73

Harmony of the Sun and the Moon

शुक्रं चन्द्रेण संयुक्तं रजः सूर्येण संयुतम् ।

तयोः समरसैकत्वं यो जानाति स योगवित् ॥७४॥

śukram candreṇa saṃyuktaṃ rajaḥ sūryeṇa saṃyutam /

tayoḥ samarasaikatvaṃ yo jānāti sa yogavit //74//

Śukra is joined with the moon. *Raja* is joined with the sun. Those who know their harmonious unity are knowers of yoga. -1.74

शोधनं नाडिजालस्य चालनं चन्द्रसूर्ययोः ।

रसानां शोषणं चैव महामुद्राभिधीयते ॥७५॥

śodhanaṃ nāḍijālasya cālanaṃ candrasūryayoḥ /

rasānām śoṣaṇam caiva mahāmudrābhidhīyate //75//

The purification of *nāḍijāla* (the *prānic* channels), the activation of *candrasūrya* (the moon and the sun), and the drying up of liquids (from the body) is called *mahāmudrā*. -1.75

Descriptions of Bandhas

उड्डीनं कुरुते यस्मादविश्रान्तं महाखगः ।

उड्डीयानं तदेव स्यान्मृत्युमातङ्गकेशरी ॥७६॥

uḍḍīnam kurute yasmādaviśrāntam mahākhagaḥ /

uḍḍīyānam tadeva syānmṛtyumātaṅgakeśarī //76//

Just like a great bird that flies upward tirelessly, one's practice of *uḍḍīyāna* bandha becomes a lion of immortality over the elephant of death. -1.76

Uḍḍīyāna Bandha

उदरात्पश्चिमे भागे अधो नाभेर्निगद्यते ।

उड्डीयानो ह्यं बन्धस्तत्र बन्धो निगद्यते ॥७७॥

udarātpaścime bhāge adho nābhernigadyate /

uḍḍīyāno hyam bandhastatra bandho nigadyate //77//

It is said that this *bandha* (lock) practice engages the area below the navel, and the back part of the abdomen. This is where it is said that the *bandha uḍḍīyāna* should be performed. -1.77

Jālandhara Bandha

बध्नाति हि सिरोजालं नाधो याति नभोजलम् ।

ततो जालन्धरो बन्धो कण्ठदुःखौघनाशनः ॥७८॥

badhnāti hi sirojālam nādho yāti nabhojalam /

tato jālandharo bandho kaṇṭhaduḥkhaughanāśanaḥ //78//

Jālandhara bandha (the throat lock) certainly blocks *sirājāla* (the network of *prānic* channels in the throat) so that *jala* (the water, meaning nectar) from *nabha* (the sky, i.e. moon) does not trickle down (into the sun). Therefore, it removes a multitude of diseases of the throat. -1.78

जालन्धरे कृते बन्धे कण्ठसंकोचलक्षणे ।

पीयूषं न पतत्यग्नौ न च वायुः प्रकुप्यति ॥७९॥

jālandhare kṛte bandhe kaṇṭhasaṅkocalakṣaṇe /

pīyūṣaṃ na patatyagnau na ca vāyuḥ prakupyati //79//

When *jālandhara bandha* is performed, as characterized (practiced) by the contraction of the throat, the nectar neither falls into the fire, nor is *vāyu* (the air, i.e. 'prāṇa') disturbed. -1.79

Mūlabandha

पार्ष्णिभागेनसंपीड्य योनिमाकुञ्चयेद्गुदम् ।

अपानमूर्ध्वमाकृष्य मूलबन्धो विधीयते ॥८०॥

pārṣṇibhāgenasampīḍya yonimākuñcayedgudam /

apānamūrdhvamākṛṣya mūlabandho vidhīyate //80//

One should press the left heel against the perineum and contract the anus while pulling the *apāna* (*vāyu*) upward. This is called *mūlabandha* (the perineum lock). -1.80

अपानप्राणयोरैक्यात् क्षयोमूत्रपुरीषयोः ।

युवा भवति वृद्धोऽपि सततं मूलबन्धनात् ॥८१॥

apānaprāṇayoraikyāt kṣayo mūtrapurīṣayoḥ /

yuvā bhavati vṛddho'pi satataṃ mūlabandhanāt //81//

Through the union of the *apāna* and *prāṇa*, urine and excrement are decreased. Even the elderly become young by continuously practicing *mūla bandha*. -1.81

Practice of Praṇava

पद्मासनं समारुह्य समकायशिरोधरः ।

नासाग्रदृष्टिरेकान्ते जपेदोङ्कारमव्ययम् ॥८२॥

padmāsanaṃ samāruhya samakāyaśirodharaḥ /

nāsāgradṛṣṭirekānte japedoṅkāramavyayam //82//

After assuming the lotus posture and maintaining *samakāyaśira* (the body and head straight) with *nāsāagradṛṣṭi* (*nāsā agra dṛṣṭi* literally, nostrils, frontal, sight - the sight fixed on the tip of the nose), one should repeat the eternal sound *Om* in *ekānta* (a secluded place). -1.82

भूर्भुवः स्वरिमे लोकाः सोमसूर्याग्निदेवताः ।

यस्या मात्रासु तिष्ठन्ति तत्परं ज्योतिरोमिति ॥८३॥

bhūrbhuvaḥ svarime lokāḥ somasūryāgnidevatāḥ /

yasyā mātrāsu tiṣṭhanti tatparaṃ jyotiromiti //83//

Om is the Supreme Light. In its *mātrā* (metre) abides the three deities of the moon, the sun, and the fire, and the three worlds indicated by the words *bhūḥ*, *bhuvaḥ* and *svaḥ*. -1.83

त्रयः कालास्त्रयो वेदास्त्रयो लोकास्त्रयः स्वराः ।

त्रयो देवाः स्थिता यत्र तत्परं ज्योतिरोमिति ॥८४॥

trayaḥ kālāstrayo vedāstrayo lokāstrayaḥ svarāḥ /

trayo devāḥ sthitā yatra tatparaṃ jyotiromiti //84//

That Supreme Light is *Om*. Therein abide the three times (past, present and future), the three *Vedas* (*Rigveda*, *Yajurveda* and *Sāmaveda*), the three worlds (*bhūḥ*, *bhuvaḥ* and *svaḥ*), the three syllables (*A*, *U* and *M*) and the three deities (*Brahmā*, *Viṣṇu* and *Maheśvara*. -1.84

क्रिया इच्छा तथा ज्ञानां ब्राह्मी रौद्री च वैष्णवी ।

त्रिधा शक्तिः स्थिता यत्र तत्परं ज्योतिरोमिति ।।८५।।

kriyā icchā tathā jñānāṃ brāhmī raudrī ca vaiṣṇavī /

tridhā śaktiḥ sthitā yatra tatparaṃ jyotiromiti //85//

That Supreme Light is *Om*, wherein abides the threefold *śaktis* (the creative powers) which are *kriyā*, *icchā* and *jñāna* (action, will and knowledge) and *Brāhmī*, *Raudrī* and *Vaiṣṇavī*. -1.85

आकाराश्च उकारश्च मकारो बिन्दुसंज्ञकः ।

त्रिधा मात्राः स्थिता यत्र तत् परं ज्योतिरोमिति ।।८६।।

ākārāśca ukārāśca makāro bindusaṅjñakaḥ /

tridhā mātrāḥ sthitā yatra tatparaṃ jyotiromiti //86//

The Supreme Light is *Om*, where the three types of letters are situated−the syllable *A*, the syllable *U*, and the syllable *M*−which is known as *bindu*. -1.86

वचसा तज्जयेद् बीजं वपुषा तत् समभ्यसेत् ।

मनसा तत्स्मरेन्नित्यं तत्परं ज्योतिरोमिति ।।८७।।

vacasā tajjaped bījaṃ vapuṣā tat samabhyaset /

manasā tatsmarennityaṃ tatparaṃ jyotiromiti //87//

That Supreme Light is *Om*. One should always recite its *bīja* (the seed syllable) orally, practice it properly with the body, and remember it in the mind. -1.87

शुचिर्वाप्यशुचिर्वापि योजपेत् प्रणवं सदा ।

न स लिप्यति पापेन पद्मपत्रमिवाम्भसा ।।८८।।

śucirvāpyaśucirvāpi yojapet praṇavaṃ sadā /

na sa lipyati pāpena padmapatramivāmbhasā //88//

One who constantly recites *pranava* (i.e. *Om*), whether one is in a pure or impure state, is not besmeared by sins, just like a lotus leaf which is not tainted by (unclean) water. -1.88

Practice of Breath Control

चले वाते चलो बिन्दुर्निश्चले निश्चलो भवेत् ।

योगी स्थाणुत्वमाप्नोति ततो वायुं निरोधयेत् ॥८९॥

cale vāte calo bindurniścale niścalo bhavet /

yogī sthāṇutvamāpnoti tato vāyuṃ nirodhayet //89//

When *vāta* (the life force) is active, the *bindu* (semen) also becomes active, and when it (the *vāta*) is stable, the *bindu* also becomes still. Therefore, a yogī wishing to obtain pillar-like steadiness should restrain the *vāyu* (the life force). -1.89

यावद् वायुः स्थितो देहे ताबज्जीवं न मुन्नति ।

मरणं तस्य निष्क्रान्तिस्ततो वायुं निरोधयेत् ॥९०॥

yāvadvāyuḥ sthito dehe tāvajjīvaṃ na muñcati /

maraṇaṃ tasya niṣkrāntistato vāyuṃ nirodhayet //90//

As long as *vāyu* (the *prāna*) remains in the body, it is called life. Its departure from the body is death. Therefore, one should restrain the *vāyu* (the life force). -1.90

यावद् बद्धो मरुद् देहे यावच्चित्तं निरामयम् ।

यावद् दृष्टिर्भुवोर्मध्ये तावत्कालभयं कुतः ॥९१॥

yāvadbaddho maruddehe yāvaccittaṃ nirāmayam /

yāvaddṛṣṭirbhruvormadhye tāvatkālabhayaṃ kutaḥ //91//

So long as *maruta* (the life force) is restrained in the body, the mind becomes *nirāmaya* (pure, free from diseases). So long as the gaze is fixed between the two eyebrows, how can there be fear of death? -1.91

अतः कालभयाद् ब्रह्मा प्राणायामपरायणः ।
योगिनो मुनयश्चैव ततो वायुं निरोधयेत् ॥९२॥

ataḥ kālabhayād brahmā prāṇāyāmaparāyaṇaḥ /

yogino munayaścaiva tato vāyuṃ nirodhayet //92//

This is why, due to the fear of death, even *Brahmā* (the Creator) is devoted to the practice of *prāṇāyāma* (the restraint of the life force). The yogīs and sages also do so. Therefore, one should restrain the *vāyu*. -1.92

Haṃsa Form of Prānāpāna Vāyu

षट्त्रिंशदङ्गुलो हंसः प्रयाणं कुरुते बहिः ।
वामदक्षिणमार्गेण ततः प्राणोऽभिधीयते ॥९३॥

ṣaṭtriṃśadaṅgulo haṃsaḥ prayāṇaṃ kurute bahiḥ /

vāmadakṣiṇamārgeṇa tataḥ prāṇo'bhidhīyate //93//

The *prayāṇa* (departure) of the *haṃsa* is of thirty-six fingers distance through the left and right pathways. Therefore, it is called *prāṇa* (the life force). -1.93

शुद्धिमेति यदा सर्वं नाडीचक्रं मलाकुलम् ।
तदैव जायते योगी प्राणसंग्रहणे क्षमः ॥९४॥

śuddhimeti yadā sarvaṃ nāḍīcakraṃ malākulam /

tadaiva jāyate yogī prāṇasaṅgrahaṇe kṣamaḥ //94//

When the *prānic* pathways and *cakras*, which are filled with impurities, are purified, then the yogī acquires the ability of *prāṇa saṅgrahaṇa* (accumulation of the life force). -1.94

Nādi Śodhana Prānāyāma

बद्धपद्मासनो योगी प्राणं चन्द्रेण पूरयेत् ।
धारयित्वा यथाशक्तिभूयः सूर्येण रेचयेत् ॥९५॥

baddhapadmāsano yogī prāṇam candreṇa pūrayet /

dhārayitvā yathāśakti bhūyaḥ sūryeṇa recayet //95//

A yogī in his *baddha padma āsana* (bound lotus posture) should fill in the *prāṇa* (life force) through *candra* (the moon, meaning the left nostril). Then holding it according to his capacity, he should expel it again through *sūrya* (the sun, meaning the right nostril). -1.95

अमृतंदधिसङ्काशं गोक्षीरधवलोपमम् ।
ध्यात्वा चन्द्रमसो बिम्बं प्राणायामी सुखी भवेत् ॥९६॥

amṛtadadhisaṅkāśam gokṣīradhavalopamam /

dhyātvā candramaso himham prāṇāyāmī sukhī bhavet //96//

A yogī who, after meditating on the disk of moon--the nectar of immortality which has the appearance (color) of curd or cow's milk or silver--practices *prāṇāyāma* (restraint of the life force/breath) will become happy. -1.96

Iḍa and Piṅgalā Prāṇāyāma

दक्षिणे श्वासमाकृष्य पूरयेदुत्तरं शनैः ।
कुम्भयित्वा विधानेन पुनश्चन्द्रेण रेचयेत् ॥९७॥

dakṣiṇeśvāsamākṛṣya pūrayeduttaram śanaiḥ /

kumbhayitvā vidhānena punaścandreṇa recayet //97//

Having drawn *śvāsa* (the breath) in through *dakṣiṇa* (the right nostril), one should slowly fill up *udara* (the abdomen). Having retained the breath using the proper method, one should expel it again through the left nostril. -1.97

प्रज्वलज्ज्वलनज्वालापुञ्जमादित्यमण्डलम् ।
ध्यात्वा नाभिस्थितं योगी प्राणायामे सुखी भवेत् ॥९८॥

prajvalajjvalanajvālāpuñjamādityamaṇḍalam /

dhyātvā nābhisthitaṃ yogī prāṇāyāmi sukhī bhavet //98//

The yogī who, after meditating on the solar disk which is a mass of brightly burning flames located at the navel, practices *prāṇāyāma* (restraint of life force/breath), will become happy. -1.98

प्राणंश्चेदिडया पिबेत्परिमितं भूयोऽन्यया रेचयेत्
पीत्वा पिङ्गलया समीरणमथो बद्ध्वा त्यजेद् वामया ।
सूर्यचन्द्रमसोरनेन विधिना बिम्बद्वयं ध्यायतां
शुद्धा नाडिगणा भवन्ति यमिनां मासत्रयादूर्ध्वतः ॥९९॥

prāṇaścediḍayā pibetparimitaṃ bhūyo'nyayā recayet

pītvā piṅgalayā samīraṇamatho baddhvā tyajed vāmayā /

sūryacandramasoranena vidhinā bimbadvayaṃ dhyāyatāṃ

śuddhā nāḍigaṇā bhavanti yamināṃ māsatrayādūrdhvataḥ //99//

When the breath is drawn in through *iḍa* (the left nostril), one should expel it again through the other (right/opposite nostril). After drawing in the air through *piṅgalā* (the right nostril), one should, after retaining it (inside), release it again through the left nostril. By meditating on the two disks of the sun and the moon according to the prescribed rules, the multitudes of *prānic* pathways become pure after three months. -1.99

The Results of Nādi Śodhana

यथेष्टं धारणं वायोरनलस्य प्रदीपनम् ।
नादाभिव्यक्तिरारोग्यं जायते नाडिशोधने ॥१००॥

yatheṣṭaṃ dhāraṇaṃ vāyoranalasya pradīpanam /

nādābhivyaktirārogyaṃ jāyate nāḍiśodhane //100//

By retaining *vāyu* (the life force) in a comfortable way, the digestive fire is ignited and *nāda* (the subtle mystical sound) becomes manifest through the purification of *nāḍis* (the subtle channels) and one attains *ārogya* (good health, a disease free state). -1.100

इति गोरक्षयोगशस्त्रे पूर्व शतकम् ।।

iti gorakṣayogaśastre pūrva śatakam //

Thus ends the First Part of *Gorakṣa Yogaśāstra.*

Uttara Śatakam

उत्तर शतकम्

Part Two

Description of Prāṇāyāma

प्राणो देहे स्थितो वायुरपानस्य निरोधनात् ।
एकश्वसनमात्रेणोद्घाटयेत् गगने गतिम् ॥१॥

prāṇo dehe sthito vāyurapānasya nirodhanāt /

ekaśvasanamātreṇodghāṭayet gagane gatim //1//

A yogī should open his way to *gagana* (space or the sky) with a single breath, through the restraint of the *prāṇa vāyu* and *apāna vāyu* that remain in the body. -2.1

रेचकः पूरकश्चैव कुम्भकः प्रणवात्मकः ।
प्राणायामो भवेत् त्रेधा मत्रद्वादशसंयुतः ॥२॥

recakaḥ pūrakaścaiva kumbhakaḥ praṇavātmakaḥ /

prāṇāyāmo bhavet tredhā mātrādvādaśasaṃyutaḥ //2//

Prāṇāyāma has three parts. They are *recaka, pūraka* and *kumbhaka* (exhalation, inhalation and retention) in combination with *praṇava* (*Om*) with twelve *mātrās* (measures). -2.2

मात्राद्वादशसंयुक्तौ दिवाकरनिशाकरौ ।

दोषजालमपघ्नन्तौ ज्ञातव्यौ योगिभिः सदा ।।३।।

mātrādvādaśasaṃyuktau divākaraniśākarau /

doṣajālamapaghnantau jñātavyau yogibhiḥ sadā //3//

The sun and moon (i.e. the *prāna* and *apāna*) should be combined with the twelve *mātrās* (measures, i.e. 12 OMs). Through this practice, all *doṣas* (physical disorders, diseases) are destroyed. The yogīs should always know these two (facts). -2.3

Three Types of Prāṇāyāma

पूरके द्वादशीकुर्यात्कुम्भके षोडशी भवेत् ।

रेचके दश ॐकराः प्राणायामः स उच्यते ।।४।।

pūrake dvādaśīkuryātkumbhake ṣoḍaśī bhavet /

recake daśa omkārāḥ prāṇāyāmaḥ sa ucyate //4//

One should inhale the breath for twelve *mātrās* (i.e. a count of twelve *Oms*), then retain it for sixteen *mātrās*, and then exhale for ten *mātrās*. This is called *prāṇāyāma* (the restraint of life force). -2.4

प्रथमे द्वादशी मात्रा मध्यमेद्विगुणा मता ।

उत्तमे त्रिगुणा प्राणायामस्य निर्णयः ।।५।।

prathame dvādaśī mātrā madhyame dviguṇā matā /

uttame triguṇā proktā prāṇāyāmasya nirṇayaḥ //5//

In the beginning one should practice using twelve *mātrās*; in the middle stage the *mātrās* should be doubled (i.e. twenty-four); in the highest stage it should be tripled (i.e. thirty-six *mātrās*) as decided for (the practice of) *prāṇāyāma*. -2.5

अधमे चोद्यते घर्मः कम्पो भवति मध्यमे ।

उत्तिष्ठत्युत्तमे योगि ततो वायुं निरोधयेत् ।।६।।

adhame codyate gharmaḥ kampo bhavati madhyame /

uttiṣṭhatyuttame yogī tato vāyuṃ nirodhayet //6//

In the lower stage of *prāṇāyāma*, there is sweating; in the middle stage there is trembling; in the highest stage the yogī rises from the ground. Therefore, he should restrain *vāyu* (the life force). -2.6

Methods of Prāṇāyāma

बद्ध पद्मासनो योगी नमस्कृत्य गुरुं शिवम् ।

भ्रूमध्ये दृष्टिरेकाकी प्राणायामं समभ्यसेत् ।।७।।

baddhapadmāsano yogī namaskṛtya guruṃ śivam /

bhrūmadhye dṛṣṭirekākī prāṇāyāmaṃ samabhyset //7//

A yogī, bound in *padmāsana*, after saluting his *Guru* and *Śiva*, should practice *prāṇāyāma* with his gaze fixed on the middle of the eyebrows. -2.7

ऊर्ध्वमाकृष्य चापानवायुं प्राणे नियोजयेत् ।

उर्ध्वमानीयते शक्त्या सर्वपापैः प्रमुच्यते ।।८।।

ūrdhvamākṛṣya cāpānavāyuṃ prāṇe niyojayet /

urdhvamānīyate śaktyā sarvapāpaiḥ pramucyate //8//

Raising the *apāna vāyu* upward, he should unite it with the *prāṇa*. When it (*apāna vāyu*) is taken upward along with *Śakti*, he is freed from all sins. -2.8

Kumbhaka Prāṇāyāma

द्वाराणां नवकं निरुद्ध्य मरुत पीत्वा दृढं धारितं

नीत्वाकाशमपानवह्निसहितं शक्त्या समुच्चालितम् ।

आत्मस्थानयुतस्त्वनेन विधिवद् विन्यस्यमूर्घ्निं ध्रुवं

यावत्तिष्ठति तावदेव महतां संघेन संस्तूयते ॥९॥

dvārāṇāṃ navakaṃ niruddhya maruta pītvā dṛḍhaṃ dhāritaṃ

nītvākāśamapānavahnisahitaṃ śaktyā samuccālitam /

ātmasthānayutastvanena vidhivad vinyasyamūrghniṃ dhruvam

yāvattiṣṭhati tāvadeva mahatāṃ saṃghena saṃstūyate //9//

After closing the nine outlets of the body, one should drink *maruta* (i.e. air) and hold it firmly. Using the *apāna vāyu* and the fire, one should correctly awaken the *Śakti*, and then unite it at the heart space. One should then certainly raise it to the head (i.e. at the *ājñā cakra*) as per the prescribed rule. The yogī who meditates on the *Ātmā* in this way, as long as one remains alive in this world, will be highly praised by the association of the great yogīs. -2.9

Results of Pranayama

प्राणायामो भवत्येवं पातकेन्धनपावकः ।

भवोदधिमहासेतुः प्रोच्यते योगिभिः सदा ॥ १० ॥

prāṇāyāmo bhavatyevaṃ pātakendhanapāvakaḥ /

bhavodadhimahāsetuḥ procyate yogibhiḥ sadā //10//

Hence, yogīs always say that *prāṇāyāma* is the fire that burns down the fuel of offences, and is a *mahāsetu* (the great bridge) which helps one get across *bhava udadhi* (the ocean of worldly existence). -2.10

आसनेन रुजो हन्ति प्राणायामेन पातकम् ।

विकारं मानसं योगी प्रत्याहारेण मुञ्चति ॥११॥

āsanena rujo hanti prāṇāyāmena pātakam /

vikāraṃ mānasaṃ yogī pratyāhāreṇa muñcati //11//

By practicing postures, diseases (of the body) are removed; through *prāṇāyāma* (restraint of the life force), offences are destroyed. Through *pratyāhāra* (withdrawal of the senses from external stimuli) the yogī releases his *mānasa vikāra* (mental modifications). -2.11

धारणाभिमतो धैर्यं ध्यानाच्चैतन्यमद्भुतम् ।

समाधौ मोक्षमानोति त्यक्त्व कर्म शुभाशुभम् ॥१२॥

dhāraṇābhimato dhairyaṃ dhyānāccaitanyamadbhutam /

samādhau mokṣamāpnoti tyaktvā karma śubhāśubham //12//

The practice of concentration as desired increases *dhairya* (patience) and through practice of *dhyāna* (meditation) a wonderful state of consciousness is attained. In *samādhi* (the superconscious state of mind), having renounced all auspicious and inauspicious karmas (actions), one attains liberation. -2.12

प्राणायामद्विषटकेन प्रत्याहारः प्रकीर्तितः ।

प्रत्याहारद्विषट्केन ज्ञायते धारणा शुभा ॥ १३॥

prāṇāyāmadviṣaṭakena pratyāhāraḥ prakīrtitaḥ /

pratyāhāradviṣaṭkena jñāyate dhāraṇā śubhā //13//

Pratyāhāra (withdrawal of the senses from external stimuli) is said to occur with twice six (twelve) *prāṇāyāmas*. *Śubha dhāraṇā* (auspicious concentration) occurs with twice six (twelve) *pratyāhāras* (one hundred forty-four *prāṇāyāmas*). -2.13

धारणा द्वादश प्रोक्ता ध्यानाद् धानविशारदैः ।

ध्यानद्वादशकेनैव समाधिरभिधीयते ॥१४॥

dhāraṇā dvādaśa proktā dhyānād dhyānaviśāradaiḥ /

dhyānadvādaśakenaiva samādhirabhidhīyate //14//

The state of *dhyāna* is attained with twelve *dhāraṇās* (one thousand seven hundred twenty-eight *prāṇāyāmas*) according to the experts in *dhyāna* (meditation). It is said that the state of *samādhi* is achieved with twelve *dhyānas* (twenty thousand seven hundred thirty-six *prāṇāyāmas*) -2.14

The Nature of Samādhi

यत्समाधौ परं ज्योतिरनन्तं विश्वमोमुखम् ।

तस्मिन् दृष्टे क्रिया कर्म यातायातं न विद्यते ॥१५॥

yatsamādhau param jyotiranantam viśvatomukham /

tasmin dṛṣṭe kriyā karma yātāyatam na vidyate //15//

One who sees in *samādhi* (the superconscious state of mind) *Parama Jyoti Ananta* (the Supreme Light Infinite) having faces all around, there does not exist any activities, any effects of past karmas, and going and coming (rounds of deaths and births) for him. -2.15

सम्बद्धासनमेढ्रमंध्रियुगलं   कर्णाक्षिनासापुटा

द्वाराण्यगुलिभिर्नियम्य पवनं वक्त्रेण सम्पूरितम् ।

ध्यात्वा वक्षसि वह्न्यपानसहितं मूर्ध्नि स्थितं धारये

देवं याति विशेषतत्त्वसमतां योगीश्वरस्तन्मयः ॥१६॥

sambaddhāsanamedhramamdhriyugalam karṇākṣināsāpuṭād

dvārāṇyagulibhirniyamya pavanam vaktreṇa sampūritam /

dhyātvā vakṣasi vahnyapānasahitam mūrdhni sthitam dhāraye

devam yāti viśeṣatattvasamatām yogīśvarastanmayaḥ //16//

After performing the posture (preferably, *siddhāsana*) one should close the openings of the ears (with the thumbs), eyes (with the index fingers), the nasal passages (with middle fingers) and mouth (with ring and little fingers) and should inhale the air through the mouth. After concentrating the *prana* in the chest along with *agni* (the fire in the abdomen) and the *apāna* (in the *mūladhāra*), he should hold them firmly in the crown of the head (*sahasrāra cakra*). In this way, the *Yogīśvara* (lord of the yogīs) absorbed in *samādhi* comes to attain *samatā* (equality or equanimity) with *Viśeṣa Tattva* (the Ultimate Reality). -2.16

The Signs of Yogasiddhi

गगनं पवने प्राप्त ध्वनिरुत्पद्यते महान् ।

घण्टादीनां प्रवाद्यानां तदा सिद्धिरदूरतः ॥१७॥

gaganaṃ pavane prāpte dhvanirutpadyate mahān /

ghaṇṭādīnāṃ pravādyānāṃ tadā siddhiradūrataḥ //17//

When the air reaches *gagana* (the sky or space, meaning *sahasrāra*), a great sound is produced similar to musical instruments such as a bell. Then (it should be known that) *siddhi* (perfection) is not far away. -2.17

प्राणायामेन युक्तेन सर्वरोक्षयो भवेत् ।

आयुक्ताभ्यासयोगेन सर्वरोगस्य संभवः ॥१८॥

prāṇāyāmena yuktena sarvarokṣayo bhavet /

ayuktābhyāsamyogena sarvarogasya sambhavaḥ //18//

Through the proper practice of *prāṇāyāma* all kinds of diseases are destroyed. Through the improper practice of yoga all types of diseases are generated. -2.18

Destruction of Diseases by Prāṇāyāma

हिक्का कासस्तथा श्वासः शिरः कर्णाक्षिवेदनाः ।

भवन्ति विविधा रोगा पवनस्य व्यतिक्रमात् ॥१९॥

hikkā kāsastathā śvāsaḥ śiraḥ karṇākṣivedanāḥ /

bhavanti vividhā rogā pavanasya vyatikramāt //19//

Various disorders like hiccups, cough, asthma, and aching of the head, ears, and eyes are caused through *vyatikrama* (the malpractice) of *pavana* (the air or life force). -2.19

यथा सिंहो गजो व्याघ्रो भवेद्वश्यः शनैः शनैः ।

अन्यथा हन्ति योक्तारं तथा वायुरसेवितः ।।२०।।

yathā siṃho gajo vyāghro bhavedvaśyaḥ śanaiḥ śanaiḥ /

anyathā hanti yoktāraṃ tathā vāyurasevitaḥ //20//

The lion, the elephant, and the tiger are brought under control slowly and slowly; otherwise, they may kill the trainer. Similarly, the improper use and practice of *pavana* (the air or life force) is detrimental. -2.20

युक्तं युक्तं त्यजेद्वायुं युक्तं युक्तं च पूरयेत् ।

युक्तं युक्तं च बध्नीयादेवं सिद्धिरदूरतः ।।२१।।

yuktaṃ yuktaṃ tyajedvāyuṃ yuktaṃ yuktaṃ ca pūrayet /

yuktaṃ yuktaṃ ca badhnīyādevaṃ siddhiradūrataḥ //21//

One should exhale the air slowly and gently, and should also inhale slowly and gently. Also, one should hold the breath slowly and gently. Thus, through such practice *siddhi* (the perfection) is near. -2.21

Description of Pratyāhāra

चरतां चक्षुरादीनां विषयेषु यथाक्रमम् ।

यत्प्रत्याहरणं तेषां प्रत्याहारः स उच्यते ।।२२।।

caratāṃ cakṣurādīnāṃ viṣayeṣu yathākramam /

yatpratyāharaṇam teṣāṃ pratyāhāraḥ sa ucyate //22//

The eyes and other senses wander towards their respective sense-objects. Their withdrawal from such (sense-objects) is called *pratyāhāra* (the withdrawal of senses). -2.22

Three Divisions of the Day

यथा तृतीयकालस्थो रविः प्रत्याहरेत्प्रभाम् ।
तृतौयाङ्गस्थितो योगी विकारं मानसं तथा ॥२३॥

yathā tṛtīyakālastho raviḥ pratyāharetprabhām /

tṛtauyāṅgasthito yogī vikāraṃ mānasaṃ tathā //23//

Just like the sun reaching the third quarter of the day withdraws its luster, so the yogī established in the third limb of yoga should withdraw his mind from its *vikāras* (mental modifications). -2.23

अङ्गमध्ये यथाङ्गान् कूर्मः संकोचयेद् ध्रुवम् ।
योगी प्रत्याहरेदेवमिन्द्रियाणि तथात्मनि ॥२४॥

aṅgamadhye yathāṅgān kūrmaḥ saṅkocayed dhruvam /

yogī pratyāharedevamindriyāṇi tathātmani //24//

Like a tortoise contracts its limbs into the middle of its shell, so the yogī should withdraw his senses from their respective sense-objects within himself. -2.24

Pratyāhāra of Likes and Dislikes

यं यं शृणोति कर्णाभ्यामप्रियं प्रियमेव वा ।
तं तमात्मेति विज्ञाय प्रत्याहरति योगवित् ॥२५॥

yaṃ yaṃ śṛṇoti karṇābhyāmapriyaṃ priyameva vā /

taṃ tamātmeti vijñāya pratyāharati yogavit //25//

Whatever he hears with his ears, whether it is pleasant or unpleasant, knowing that it is *Ātmā* (the Self), the expert in yoga withdraws himself from hearing. -2.25

अगन्धमथवा गन्धं यं यं जिघ्रति नासिका ।
तं तमात्मेति विज्ञाय प्रत्याहरति योगवित ॥२६॥

agandhamathavā gandhaṃ yaṃ yaṃ jighrati nāsikā /

taṃ tamātmeti vijñāya pratyāharati yogavit //26//

Whatever he smells with his nose, whether fragrant or stinking, knowing that it is *Ātmā* (the Self), the expert in yoga withdraws himself from smelling. -2.26

अमेध्यमथवा मेध्यं यं यं पश्यति चक्षुषा ।
तं तमात्मेति विज्ञाय प्रत्याहरति योगवित ॥२७॥

amedhyamathavā medhyaṃ yaṃ yaṃ paśyati cakṣuṣā /

taṃ tamātmeti vijñāya pratyāharati yogavita //27//

Whatever he sees with his eyes, whether pure or impure, knowing that it is *Ātmā* (the Self), the expert in yoga withdraws himself from seeing or sight -2.27

अस्पृश्यमथवा स्पृश्यं यं यं स्पृशति चर्मणा ॥
तं तमात्मेति विज्ञाय प्रत्याहरति योगवित ॥२८॥

aspṛśyamathavā spṛśyaṃ yaṃ yaṃ spṛśati carmaṇā /

taṃ tamātmeti vijñāya pratyāharati yogavit //28//

Whatever he senses with his skin, whether perceptible or not perceptible, knowing that it is *Ātmā* (the Self), the expert in yoga withdraws himself from his sense of touch. -2.28

लावण्यमलावण्यं वा यं यं रसति जिह्वया ।
तं तमात्मेति विज्ञाय प्रत्याहरति योगवित् ॥२९॥

lāvaṇyamalāvaṇyaṃ vā yaṃ yaṃ rasati jihvayā /

taṃ tamātmeti vijñāya pratyāharati yogavit //29//

Whatever he tastes with his tongue, whether salty or not salty, knowing that it is *Ātmā* (the Self), the expert in yoga withdraws himself from his sense of taste. -2.29

Pratyāhāra of the Nectar

चन्द्रामृत्मयीं धारां प्रत्याहरति भास्करः ।

यत्प्रत्यहरणं तस्याः प्रत्याहारः स उच्यते ।।३०।।

candrāmṛtmayīṃ dhārāṃ pratyāharati bhāskaraḥ /

yatpratyāharaṇaṃ tasyāḥ pratyāhāraḥ sa ucyate //30//

The sun devours (withdraws) *dhārā* (the fountain) full of *amṛta* (the nectar) from the moon. One should drink that shower of the nectar, withdrawing it back from the sun. That is called *pratyāhāra* (in the sense of taking the shower of *amṛta* back). -2.30

एकस्त्री भुज्यते द्वाभ्यामागता चन्द्रमण्डलात् ।

तृतीयो यः पुनस्ताभ्यां स भवेदजरामरः ।।३१।।

ekastrī bhujyate dvābhyāmāgatā candramaṇḍalāt /

tṛtīyo yaḥ punastābhyāṃ sa bhavedajarāmaraḥ //31//

There is one female (meaning the fountain of *amṛta*) that comes from the lunar region to be enjoyed by two (the sun and the moon). If the third one enjoys her, he becomes free from old age and death. -2.31

Viparītakaraṇi Mudrā

नाभिदेशे वसत्येको भास्करो दहनात्मनः ।

अमृतात्मा स्थितो नित्यं तालुमूले च चन्द्रमाः ।।३२।।

nābhideśe vasatyeko bhāskaro dahanātmanaḥ /

amṛtātmā sthito nityaṃ tālumūle ca candramāḥ //32//

The one sun dwells in the region of the navel in the form or spirit of fire. The moon in the form or spirit of nectar is always located at *tālumūla* (at the root of the palate). -2.32

वर्षत्यधोमुखश्चन्द्रो ग्रस्त्यूर्ध्वमुखो रविः ।

ज्ञातव्या करणी तत्र यथा पीयूषमाप्यते ।।३३।।

varṣatyadhomukhaścandro grastyūrdhvamukho raviḥ /

jñātavyā karaṇī tatra yathā pīyūṣamāpyate //33//

The downward facing moon drops down the nectar. The upward facing sun devours that nectar (that drops down from the moon). So, one should know *karaṇi* (meaning the inverted pose) in order to get *pīyūṣa* (the nectar). -2.33

ऊर्ध्वं नाभिरधस्तालुरूर्ध्वं भानुरधः शशी ।

करणि विपरीताख्या गुरुवाक्येन लभ्यते ।।३४।।

ūrdhva nābhiradhastālurūrdhvaṃ bhānuradhaḥ śaśī /

karaṇi viparītākhyā guruvākyena labhyate //34//

While the navel is above and the palate is below, in other words, while the sun is above and the moon is below, then that is known as *viparīta karaṇi āsana* (the inverted pose). One should receive it through the instructions of a guru (teacher). -2.34

Anāhata Cakra

त्रिधा बद्धो वृषो यत्र रोरवीति महास्वनः ।

अनाहतं च तच्चक्रं हृदये योगिनो विदुः ।।३५।।

tridhā baddho vṛṣo yatra roravīti mahāsvanaḥ /

anāhataṃ ca taccakraṃ hṛdaye yogino viduḥ //35//

Whereas a bull tied up three rounds with a rope bellows in a horrific way, similarly, yogīs should know that it is in the *anāhata cakra* located at the heart where the *jīva* (the embodied Self) yells, being tied up by the snares of this illusory world. -2.35

अनाहतमतिक्रम्य चाक्रम्य मणिपूरकम् ।

प्राप्ते प्राणे महापद्मं योगी स्वयमृतायते ।। ३६।।

anāhatamatikramya cākramya maṇipūrakam /

prāpte prāṇe mahāpadmaṃ yogī svayamṛtāyate //36//

When the *prāṇa* (life force) reaches the *mahāpadma* (great lotus i.e. *sahasrāra cakra* - the thousand-petalled lotus at the crown of the head), after having gone beyond the *maṇipūra cakra* and *anāhata cakra*, the yogī by himself attains the state of *amṛtā* (immortality). -2.36

ऊर्ध्वं षोडशपत्रपद्मगलितं प्राणाद्वाप्तं हठा-

दूर्ध्वस्यो रसनां निधाय विधिवच्छक्तिं परां चिन्तयेत् ।

तत्कल्लोलकलाजलं सुविमलं जिह्वाकुलम् यः पिबे-

न्निर्दोषः समृणालकोपुर्योगी चिरं जीवति ।। ३७।।

ūrdhavaṃ ṣoḍaśapatrapadmagalitaṃ prāṇādvāptaṃ haṭhād-

ūrdhvasyo rasanāṃ nidhāya vidhivacchaktiṃ parāṃ cintayet /

tatkallolakalājalaṃ suvimalaṃ jihvākulam yaḥ pibe-

nnirdoṣaḥ samṛṇālakomalavapuryogī ciraṃ jīvati //37//

After turning his tongue upward into the cavity (of the skull) according to approved method, one should obtain the nectar forcibly by fixing it (the tongue) to the palate so that (the nectar) drops down from the sixteen-petalled lotus above, and then he should contemplate *Parāma Śakti* (the Supreme Power). That flawless yogī, who drinks the extremely pure water flowing from that lotus (mentioned above), from *kula* (the home) of his tongue, lives a long life with a body as soft as a lotus stalk. -2.37

Kāki Mudrā

काकचञ्चुवदास्येन शीतलं सलिलं पिबेत् ।

प्राणापानविधानेन योगी भवति निर्जरः ॥३८॥

kākacañcuvadāsyena śītalaṃ salilaṃ pibet /

prāṇāpānavidhānena yogī bhavati nirjaraḥ //38//

The yogī should drink the cool flow of air with the mouth formed like the beak of a crow. One does not become old by following the practice of *prāṇa* and *apāna* according to prescribed method. -2.38

रसनातालुमूलेन यः प्राणमनिलं पिबेत् ।

अब्दार्द्धेन भवेतस्य सर्वरोगस्य संक्षयः ॥३९॥

rasanātālumūlena yaḥ prāṇamanilaṃ pibet /

abdārddhena bhavetasya sarvarogasya saṃkṣayaḥ //39//

One who drinks *prāṇa* anila (meaning *vāyu*) with the tongue located at the root of the palate, their multifarious diseases are totally destroyed after half a year. -2.39

Vishuddha Cakra

विशुद्धे पञ्चमे चक्रे ध्यात्वासौ सकलामृतम् ।

उन्मार्गेण हृतं याति वञ्चयित्वा मुखं रवेः ॥४०॥

viśuddhe pañcame cakre dhyātvāsau sakalāmṛtam /

unmārgeṇa hṛtaṃ yāti vañcayitvā mukhaṃ raveḥ //40//

One who, having contemplated the nectar fully in the fifth *cakra visuddhi* (also called *viśuddha*), and having the mouth of the sun (located at the navel region) deprived of the nectar, goes to confiscate it (the nectar) through the opposite route. -2.40

विशब्देन स्मृतो हंसः नैर्मल्यं शुद्धिरुच्यते ।

अतः कण्ठे विशुद्धाख्यं चक्रं चक्रविदो विदुः ॥४१॥

viśabdena smṛto haṃsaḥ nairmalyaṃ śuddhirucyate /

ataḥ kaṇṭhe viśuddhākhyaṃ cakram cakravido viduḥ //41//

It is understood that the sound/word '*vi*' means *haṃsa* (literally, a swan that constantly goes out and comes in (here the meaning is: the breath) and it is understood that the word '*śuddhi*' means purity. Therefore, the *cakra* named '*viśuddha*' located at the throat is known well by the expert of the *cakras* in yoga. -2.41

Depriving the Mouth of the Sun

अमृतं कन्दरे कृत्वा नासान्तसुषिरे क्रमात् ।

स्वयमुच्चालितं याति वर्जयित्वा मुखं रवेः ॥४२॥

amṛtaṃ kandare kṛtvā nāsāntasuṣire kramāt /

svayamuccālitam yāti varjayitvā mukhaṃ raveḥ //42//

After one has gradually placed the nectar into the cave at the end of the nose, the *prāna*, after abandoning the mouth of the sun, goes up by itself (in its own way) into the cavity. -2.42

Drinking of the Lunar Nectar

बद्धं सोमकलाजलं सुविमलं कण्ठस्थलादूर्ध्वतो

नासान्ते सुषिरे नयेच्च गगनद्वारान्ततः सर्वतः ।

ऊर्ध्वास्यो भुवि सन्निपत्य निरामुत्तानपादः पिबे

देवं यः कुरुते जितेन्द्रियगणो नैवास्ति तस्य क्षयः ॥ ४३॥

baddhaṃ somakalājalaṃ suvimalaṃ kaṇṭhasthalādūrdhvato

nāsānte suṣire nayecca gaganadvārāntataḥ sarvataḥ /

ūrdhvāsyo bhuvi sannipatya nirāmuttānapādaḥ pibed

evaṃ yaḥ kurute jitendriyagaṇo naivāsti tasya kṣayaḥ //43//

Having stopped the extremely pure water (nectar) of the crescent moon located at the upper region of the throat, one should fill it into the cavity at the end of the nostrils. Then, closing all the gates of the *prāna*, one should inhale with *prāna* and *apāna* at the *gagana* (the crown of the head). Then, he should lie flat with extended legs on the ground and drink the nectar (mentioned above). The yogī who regularly does so in this way, and has subdued their senses, there is no destruction for them. -2.43

उर्ध्वं जिह्वां स्थिरीकृत्य सोमपनां करोति यः ।

मासार्द्धेन न सन्देहो मृत्युं जयति योगवित् ॥४४॥

urdhvaṃ jihvāṃ sthirīkṛtya somapānaṃ karoti yaḥ /

māsārddhena na sandeho mṛtyuṃ jayati yogavit //44//

One who is expert in yoga, and drinks *soma* (the nectar from the moon) by establishing his tongue upward in the cavity behind the palate, conquers death within half a month. There is no doubt about it. -2.44

बद्धम् मूलबिल येन तेन विघ्नो विदारितः ।

अजरामरमाप्रोति यथा पञ्चमुखो हरः ॥४५॥

baddhaṃ mūlabila yena tena vighno vidāritaḥ /

ajarāmaramāpnoti yathā pañcamukho haraḥ //45//

The yogī who is successful in locking the main door overcomes all obstacles and attains *ajara* and *amara* (changeless and immortal) states like *Pañcamukha* (five-faced) *Śiva*. -2.45

संपीड्य रसनाग्रेण राजदन्तबिलं महत् ।

ध्यात्वामृतमयीं देवीं षण्मासेन कविर्भवेत् ॥४६॥

saṃpīḍya rasanāgreṇa rājadantabilaṃ mahat /

dhyātvāmṛtamayīṃ devīṃ ṣaṇmāsena kavirbhavet //46//

The yogī who presses the tip of his tongue against the great cavity behind *rājadanta* (the incisor teeth) and contemplates *Amṛtamayī Devī* (the Goddess of Nectar), becomes a *kavi* (poet) within six months. -2.46

सर्वद्वाराणि बध्नाति तदूर्ध्वं धारितं महत् ।

न मुञ्चत्यमृतंकोऽपि स पन्थाः पञ्चधारणाः ॥४७॥

sarvadvārāṇi badhnāti tadūrdhvaṃ dhāritaṃ mahat /

na muñcatyamṛtaṅko'pi sa panthāḥ pañcadhāraṇāḥ //47//

When the great flow of the nectar from above is blocked with the tip of the tongue, the gates of all the *nāḍis* are closed. Due to the block of the above route, the nectar does not fall anywhere. This way of *dhāraṇā* (concentration on the nectar) is like *pañca dhāraṇā* (the five types of concentration on the five elements). -2.47

Experience of the Nectar Juice

चुम्बन्ती यदि लम्बिकाग्रमनिशं जिह्वा रसस्यन्दिनी

सक्षारं कटुकाम्लदुग्धसदृशं मध्वाज्यतुल्यं तथा ।

व्याधीनां हरणं जरान्तकरणं शास्त्राङ्गमोदगीरणं

तस्य स्यादमरत्वमष्टगुणितं सिद्धाङ्गनाकर्षणम् ॥४८॥

cumbantī yadi lambikāgramaniśaṃ jihvā rasasyandinī

sakṣāraṃ kaṭukāmladugdhasadṛśaṃ madhvājyatulyaṃ tathā /

vyādhīnāṃ haraṇaṃ jarāntakaraṇaṃ śāstrāṅgamodgīraṇam

tasya syādamaratvamaṣṭaguṇitaṃ siddhāṅganākarṣaṇam //48//

The yogi, who regularly kisses the *rasa* (the nectar) donor with the tip of his tongue, experiences its tastes as salty, pungent, sour or like milk, honey, and ghee. All diseases and old age are ended (through this practice) and that yogī comprehends and explains *śāstras* (the scriptures) and their *aṅgas* (the branches) without studying them, and achieves *amaratva* (immortality) and *aṣṭaguṇas* or *aṣṭasiddhis* (the eight supernatural powers) and attracts *siddhas* (adepts) and *aṅganā* (beautiful women). -2.48

अमृतापूर्णदेहस्य योगिनो द्वित्रिवत्सरात् ।

ऊर्ध्वं प्रवर्तते रेतोऽप्यणिमादिगुणोदयः ॥४९॥

amṛtāpūrṇadehasya yogino dvitrivatsarāt /

ūrdhvaṃ pravartate reto'pyaṇimādiguṇodayaḥ //49//

The yogī's body becomes full of the nectar after two or three years and his *reta* (semen) rises upward. Through this he attains *aṇimādiguṇas* (the *aṇimā*, etc. qualities, meaning the supernatural powers). -2.49

इन्धनानि यथा वह्निस्तैलवर्तिं च दीपकः ।

तथा सोमकलापूर्णं देहं देही न मुञ्चति ॥५०॥

īndhanāni yathā vahnistailavartiṃ ca dīpakaḥ /

tathā somakalāpūrṇaṃ dehaṃ dehī na muñcati //50//

When there is fuel, there is fire, and when there is oil and wick, there is light. Similarly, *Dehī* (the indweller of the body, the Self) does not depart *deha* (the body) of the yogī when it is *somakalāpūrṇa* (full of lunar nectar). -2.50

नित्यसोमकलपूर्णशरीरं यस्य योगिनः ।

तक्षकेणापि दष्टस्य विषं तस्य न सर्पति ॥५१॥

nityaṃ somakalāpūrṇa śarīraṃ yasya yoginaḥ /

takṣakeṇāpi daṣṭasya viṣaṃ tasya na sarpati //51//

A yogī whose body is always full of the lunar nectar, poison does not spread in his body, though a *Takṣaka* (king of serpents) itself bites him. -2.51

Description of Dhāranā

आसनेन समायुक्तः प्राणायामेन संयुतः ।

प्रत्याहारेण सम्पन्नो धारणां च समभ्यसेत् ॥५२॥

āsanena samāyuktaḥ prāṇāyāmena saṃyutaḥ /

pratyāhāreṇa sampanno dhāraṇāṃ ca samabhyaset //52//

The yogi, who is equipped with posture and breath control, and also rich in (the practice of) *pratyāhāra* (withdrawal of senses), should properly practice *dhāraṇā* (concentration). -2.52

हृदये पञ्चभूतानां धारणा च पृथक् पृथक् ।

मनसो निश्चलत्वेन धारणा साभिधीयते ॥५३॥

hṛdaye pañcabhūtānāṃ dhāraṇā ca pṛthak pṛthak /

manaso niścalatvena dhāraṇā sābhidhīyate //53//

Concentration on each *pañcabhūtā* (the five elements) in the heart with a steady mind is called *dhāraṇā* (concentration). -2.53

Dhāranā on Earth Element

य पृथ्वी हरितालहेमरुचिरा पीता लकारान्विता

संयुक्ता कमलासनेन हि चतुष्कोणाहृदि स्थायिनी ।

प्राणांस्तत्र विलीय पञ्चघटिकं चित्तान्वितान्धारये

देषा स्तम्भकरी सदाक्षितिजयं कुर्यद् भुवो धारणा ॥५४॥

yā pṛthvī haritālahemarucirā pītā lakārānvitā

saṃyuktā kamalāsanena hi catuṣkoṇāhṛdisthāyinī /

prāṇāṃstatra vilīya pañcaghaṭikaṃ cittānvitāndhārayed-

eṣāstambhakarī sadā kṣitijayaṃ kuryadbhuvo dhāraṇā //54//

The earth element has a bright yellow gold or radiant orpiment color, with a *bīja* (the seed) *'lam'* in the middle of a yellowish square altar in the heart, where the God *Brahmā* is seated in lotus pose. One should concentrate on the *'lam' bīja* (seed) and dissolve the *prāna* together with the mind there (in the heart) for five *ghaṭikā* (two hours). In this way, this *dhāranā* practice is the bestower of steadying effect (on the *prāna* and mind). One should always practice this concentration to conquer the earth. -2.54

Dhāranā on Water Element

आर्द्धेन्दुप्रतिमं च कुन्दधवलं कण्ठेऽम्बुतत्त्वं स्थितं
यत्पीयूषवकारबीजसहितं युक्तं सदा विष्णुना ।
प्राण तत्रविलीय पञ्चघटिका चित्तानिवितं धारये-
देषा दुःसहकालकूटदहनी स्याद्वारुणी धारणा ॥५५॥

ārddhendupratimaṃ ca kundadhavalaṃ

kaṇthe'mbutattvaṃ sthitaṃ

yatpīyūṣavakārabījasahitaṃ yuktaṃ sadā vikṣṇunā /

prāṇam tatravilīya pañcaghaṭikā cittānivitaṃ dhāraye-

deṣā duḥsahakālakūṭadahanī syādvāruṇī dhāraṇā //55//

Ambutattva (the water element) has the color of the crescent moon or white jasmine. Its nectar is bestowed with the *bīja* (seed) *'vam'* located at the throat, and it is always related to Lord *Viṣṇu*. One should concentrate on the *'vam' bīja* (seed) and dissolve the prāna together with the mind there (in the heart) for five *ghaṭikā* (two hours). In this way, this *dhāranā* practice is the bestower of steadying effect (on the *prāna* and mind). This is certainly *vāruṇī dhāranā* (concentration on water element) which even burns down *duḥsaha kālakūṭa* (the deadliest poison most difficult to digest or eliminate from the body). -2.55

Dhāranā on Fire Element

यत्तालुस्थितमिन्द्रगोपसदृशं तत्त्वं त्रिकोणानलं

तेजो   रेफ़युतं   प्रवालरुचिरं   सत्सङ्गतम् ।

प्राणं तत्र विलीय पञ्चघटिकं चित्तान्वितं धारये

देषा वह्निजयं सदा वितनुते वैश्वानरी धारणा ॥५६॥

yattālusthitamindragopasadṛśaṃ tattvaṃ trikoṇānalaṃ

tejo rephayutaṃ pravālaruciraṃ rudreṇa satsaṅgatam /

prāṇaṃ tatra vilīya pañcaghaṭikaṃ cittānvitaṃ dhārayed

eṣā vahnijayaṃ sadā vitanute vaiśvānarī dhāraṇā //56//

The fire element is red, similar to the cochineal insect, triangular in shape, bright like coral and magnificent with the *bīja* (seed) *'ram'* and is associated with God *Rudra*. One should concentrate on the *'ram' bīja* (seed) and dissolve the *prāna* together with the mind there in the fire element for five *ghaṭikā* (two hours). In this way, this *vaiśvānarī dhāranā* (concentration on the fire element) is perfected. This practice always brings *vahnijaya* (victory over the fire element). -2.56

Dhāranā on Air Element

यद्भिन्नाञ्जनपुञ्जसन्निभमिदं स्यूतं भ्रुवोरन्तरे

तत्त्वं   वायुमयं   यकारसहितं   तत्रेश्वरो देवता ।

प्राणं तत्रविलीय पञ्चघटिकं चित्तान्वितं धारये

देषा खेगमनं करोति यमिनः स्याद्वायवीधारणा ॥५७॥

yadbhinnāñjanapuñjasannibhamidaṃ syūtaṃ bhruvorantare

tattvaṃ vāyumayaṃ yakārasahitaṃ tatreśvaro devatā /

prāṇaṃ tatra vilīya pañcaghaṭikaṃ cittānvitaṃ dhārayed-

eṣā khegamanaṃ karoti yaminaḥ syādvāyavīdhāraṇā //57//

The air element is located between the eyebrows. It looks like the black collyrium and is associated with the *bīja* (seed) *'yam'*. Its *devatā* (deity) is *Īśvara*. One should concentrate on the *'yam' bīja* (seed) and dissolve the *prāna* together with the mind there in the air element for five *ghaṭikā* (two hours). In this way, through the practice of *vāyavī dhāranā* (concentration on the air element) the practitioner travels in space. -2.57

Dhāranā on Ether Element

आकाशं सुविशुद्धवारिसदृशं यद् ब्रह्मरन्ध्रस्थितं

तन्नादेन सदाशिवेन सहितं तत्वं हकारान्वितम् ।

प्राणं तत्र विलीया पञ्चघटीकं चित्तन्वितं धारये

देषा मोक्षकपाटपाटनपतुः प्रोक्ता नभोधारणा ॥५८॥

ākāśaṃ suviśuddhavārisadṛśaṃ yad brahmarandhrasthitaṃ

tannādena sadāśivena sahitaṃ tatvaṃ hakārānvitam /

prāṇaṃ tatra vilīyā pañcaghaṭīkaṃ cittanvitaṃ dhārayed-

eṣā mokṣakapāṭapāṭanapatuḥ proktā nabhodhāraṇā //58//

The ether element is located at the *brahma randhra* (the hole of *Brahma*) at the crown of the head, which is like perfectly pure water. It is associated with the *devatā Sadā Śiva*, *nāda* (the inner mystical sound), and the *bīja* (seed) *'ham'*. One should concentrate on the *'ham' bīja* (seed) and dissolve the *prāna* together with the mind there in the ether element for five *ghaṭikā* (two hours). In this way, through the practice of *nabhodhāranā* (concentration on the ether element) the practitioner breaks open the door to liberation. -2.58

स्तम्भिनी द्राविणी चैव दाहिनी भ्रामिणी तथा ।

शोषिणी च भवात्येषा भूतानां पञ्चधारणाः ॥५९॥

stambhinī drāviṇī caiva dāhinī bhrāmiṇī tathā /

śoṣiṇī ca bhavatyeṣā bhūtānāṃ pañcadhāraṇāḥ //59//

Concentration on the earth element is stabilizing, on the water element dissolving, on the fire element burning, on the air element mobile, and on the ether element desiccative, respectively. These are the *pañcadhāraṇā* (the five types of concentration) on the *bhūtās* (the five elements, i.e. earth, water, fire, air, ether). -2.59

कर्मणा मनसा वाचा धारणाः पञ्चदुर्लभाः ।

विज्ञान सततं योगी सर्वदुःखैः प्रमुच्यते ॥६०॥

karmaṇā manasā vācā dhāraṇāḥ pañcadurlabhāḥ /

vijñāna satataṃ yogī sarvaduḥkhaiḥ pramucyate //60//

The practice of *pañcadhāraṇā* (the five types of concentration) by action, mind and speech is rare. The yogī who acquires perpetual knowledge of *pañcadhāraṇā* (through his practice) becomes free from all types of sufferings. -2.60

Description of Dhyāna

स्मृत्येव सर्वचिन्तायां धातुरेकः प्रपद्यते ।

यच्चित्ते निर्मला चिन्ता तद्धि ध्यानं प्रचक्षते ॥६१॥

smṛtyeva sarvacintāyāṃ dhāturekaḥ prapadyate /

yaccitte nirmalā cintā taddhi dhyānaṃ pracakṣate //61//

Smṛti (memory) means constant recollection of the one *Ātmatattva* (the Self Reality) in the mind from among all thoughts. It is called meditation when there are pure thoughts in the mind. 2.61

द्विविधं भवति ध्यानं सकलं निष्कलं तथा ।

चर्याभेदेन सकलं निष्कलं निर्गुणं भवेत् ॥ ६२॥

dvividham bhavati dhyānam sakalam niṣkalam tathā /

caryābhedena sakalam niṣkalam nirguṇam bhavet //62//

Dhyāna (meditation) is of two types: *sakala* (having attributes or qualities) and *niṣkala* (without attributes or qualities). It becomes *sakala dhyāna* while one meditates on God with attributes, and it becomes *niṣkala*, or *nirguṇa dhyāna*, while one meditates on God without attributes. This difference is according to the prescribed routine/activity of meditation practice. -2.62

Elimination of Sins through Dhyāna

अन्तश्चेतो बहिश्चक्षुरधः स्थाप्य सुखासनः ।

कुण्डलिन्या समायुक्तं ध्यात्वा मुच्येत किल्विषात् ॥६३॥

antaśceto bahiścakṣuradhaḥ sthāpya sukhāsanaḥ /

kuṇḍalinyā samāyuktam dhyātvā mucyeta kilviṣāt //63//

One should perform *sukhāsana* (literally, happy or comfortable pose) with the mind internally focused and eyes externally gazing downward. Contemplating with due attention on *Kuṇḍalini*, one is freed from sins. -2.63

आधारं प्रथमं चक्रं स्वर्णाभं च चतुर्दलम् ।

कुण्डलिन्या समायुक्तं ध्यात्वा मुच्येत किल्विषैः ॥६४॥

ādhāram prathamam cakram svarṇābham ca caturdalam /

kuṇḍalinyā samāyuktam dhyātvā mucyeta kilviṣaiḥ //64//

Ādhāra is the first *cakra*, with four petals and a color similar to bright gold. Contemplating with due attention on this spot along with *Kuṇḍalini*, one is freed from all sins. -2.64

स्वाधिष्ठाने च षट्पत्रे सन्माणिक्यसमप्रभे ।

नासाग्रदृष्टिरात्मानं ध्यात्वा योगी सुखी भवेत् ॥६५॥

svādhiṣṭhāne ca ṣaṭpatre sanmāṇikyasamaprabhe /

nāsāgradṛṣṭirātmānaṃ dhyātvā yogī sukhī bhavet //65//

Svādhiṣṭhāna (literally, establishment of the Self) *cakra* has six petals and its bright color is similar to a ruby. A yogī who contemplates *Ātmā* (the Self), gazing at the tip of the nose, becomes happy. -2.65

Achievement of Strength through Dhyāna

तरुणादित्यसंकाशे चक्रे च मणिपूरते ।

नासाग्रदृष्टिरात्मानं ध्यात्वा संक्षोभयेज्जगत् ॥६६॥

taruṇādityasaṅkāśe cakre ca maṇipūrate /

nāsāgradṛṣṭirātmānaṃ dhyātvā saṅkṣobhayejjagat //66//

Maṇipūra cakra is similar to *taruṇa āditya* (literally, the adult sun or rising sun) in the sky. A yogī who contemplates on the Self at this luminous city center, gazing at the tip of the nose, shakes the whole world. -2.66

हृदाकाशे स्थितं शम्भु प्रचण्डरवितेजसम् ।

नासाग्रे दृष्टिमाधाय ध्यात्वा ब्राह्ममयो भवेत् ॥६७॥

hṛdākāśe sthitaṃ śambhu pracaṇḍaravitejasam /

nāsāgre dṛṣṭimādhāya dhyātvā brāhmamayo bhavet //67//

A yogī who contemplates on *Śambhu* (another name of *Śiva*), situated in the space of the heart, fixing the gaze at the tip of the nose, becomes assimilated into *Brahma* (the Absolute Reality). -2.67

विद्युत्प्रभे च हृदत्पद्मे प्राणायामविभेदतः ।
नासाग्रदृष्टिरात्मानं ध्यात्वा ब्रह्ममयो ।।६८।।

vidyutprabhe ca hṛdatpadme prāṇāyāmavibhedataḥ /

nāsāgradṛṣṭirātmānaṃ dhyātvā brahmamayo bhavet //68//

The *anāhata cakra* in the space of the heart is radiant like lightning. A yogī who contemplates on the space of the heart, fixing the gaze at the tip of the nose, and at the same time practicing various types of *prāṇāyāma*, becomes identical to *Brahma* (the Absolute Reality). -2.68

Immortality through Ātmā Dhyāna

सततं घणिटकामध्ये विशुद्धे दीपकप्रभे ।
नासाग्रदृष्टिरात्मानं ध्यात्वानन्दमयो भवेत् ।।६९।।

satataṃ ghaṇṭikāmadhye viśuddhe dīpakaprabhe /

nāsāgradṛṣṭirātmānaṃ dhyātvānandamayo bhavet //69//

One who constantly contemplates on the Self shining like a lamp in the middle of the throat at the *viśuddha cakra*, while fixing the gaze at the tip of the nose, becomes *ānandamaya* (blissful). -2.69

भ्रुवोरन्तर्गतं देवं सन्माणिक्यशिखोपमम् ।
नासाग्रदृष्टिरात्मानं ध्यात्वानन्दमयो भवेत् ।।७०।।

bhruvorantargataṃ devaṃ sanmāṇikyaśikhopamam /

nāsāgradṛṣṭirātmānaṃ dhyātvānandamayo bhavet //70//

The God who is located between the eyebrows looks like a true jewel on the crown. Contemplating on the Self while gazing at the tip of the nose, one becomes blissful. -2.70

ध्यायन्नीलनिभं नित्यं भ्रूमध्ये परमेश्वरम् ।
आत्मानं विजितप्राणो योगी मोक्षमवाप्नुयात् ॥७१॥

dhyāyannīlanibhaṃ nityaṃ bhrūmadhye parameśvaram /

ātmānaṃ vijitaprāṇo yogī mokṣamavāpnuyāt //71//

The yogī who always contemplates on *Nīlanibha* or *Nīlābha* (here it means one having blue color) *Parameśvara* (the Supreme Lord, i.e. *Śiva*) at the spot between the two eyebrows conquers *prāṇa* and attains *mokṣa* (liberation). -2.71

निर्गुणं च शिवं शान्तं गगने विश्वतोमुखम् ।
नासाग्रदृष्टिरेकाकी ध्वात्वा ब्रह्ममयो भवेत् ॥७२॥

nirguṇaṃ ca śivaṃ śāntaṃ gagane viśvatomukham /

nāsāgradṛṣṭirekākī dhvātvā brahmamayo bhavet //72//

While gazing at the tip of the nose, one who contemplates on the absolute, *Śiva* (benevolent), tranquil, having faces on all directions in the sky, assumes the form of the *Brahma* or becomes identical to *Brahma*. -2.72

Attainment of Liberation through Dhyāna

आकाशे यत्र शब्दः स्यात्तदाज्ञाचक्रमुच्यते ।
तत्रात्मानं शिवं ध्यात्वा योगी मुक्तिमवाप्नुयात् ॥७३॥

ākāśe yatra śabdaḥ syāttadājñācakramucyate /

tatrātmānaṃ śivaṃ dhyātvā yogī muktimavāpnuyāt //73//

Space is the place of the mind from where the mystical sound is heard. That space is called *ājñācakra* (the center of command). There in the Self, the yogī contemplating on *Śiva* obtains *mukti* (liberation). -2.73

निर्मलं गगनाकारं मरीचिजलसन्निभम् ।

आत्मानं सर्वगं ध्यात्वा योगीमुक्तिमवाप्नुयात् ।।७४।।

nirmalaṃ gaganākāraṃ marīcijalasannibham /

ātmānaṃ sarvagaṃ dhyātvā yogīmuktimavāpnuyāt //74//

The yogī, after contemplating on the Self Omnipresent, which is pure, has the shape of the sky, and glitters like mirage water, attains *mukti* (liberation). -2.74

Attainment of Siddhis through Dhyāna

गुदं मेढ्रं च नाभिश्च हृत्पद्मं च तदूर्ध्वतः ।

घण्टिका लंबिकास्थान भ्रूमध्ये च नभोबिलम् ।।७५।।

कथितानि नवैतानि ध्यानस्थानानि योगिभिः ।

उपाधितत्वमुक्तानि कुर्वन्त्यष्टगुणोदयम् ।।७६।।

gudaṃ meḍhraṃ ca nābhiśca hṛtpadmaṃ ca tadurdhvataḥ /

ghaṇṭikā lambikāsthāna bhrūmadhye ca nabhobilam //75//

kathitāni navaitāni dhyānasthānāni yogibhiḥ /

upādhitatvamuktāni kurvantyaṣṭaguṇodayam //76//

Guda (anus), *meḍhra* (penis), *nābhi* (navel), *hṛtpadma* (heart lotus), and above that (i.e. *viśuddha*, the neck center), *ghaṇṭikā* (Adam's apple), *lambikā* (uvula in the throat), *bhrūmadhya* (spot between the eyebrows) and *nabhobila* (literally, hole of the sky or cavity at the crown of the head) are nine places of meditation which are told by yogīs. They liberate one from the attributes of the senses, and emanate the eight supernatural powers/qualities. -2.75-76

एषु ब्रह्मात्मकं तेजः शिवज्योतिरनुत्तमम् ।।

ध्वात्वा ज्ञात्वा विमुक्तः स्यादिति गोरक्षभाषितम् ।।७७।।

eṣu brahmātmakaṃ tejaḥ śivajyotiraṇuttamam /

dhvātvā jñātvā vimuktaḥ syāditi gorakṣabhāṣitam //77//

The yogī, who after contemplating on those places (mentioned above) and knowing the extremely brilliant light of *Śiva*, which is illuminating and identical to *Brahma* (the Absolute), is liberated. Thus, these words are rarely spoken by *Gorakṣa*. -2.77

Kuṇḍalinī: Union with Shiva

नाभौ संयम्य पवनगतिमधो रोधयंसंप्रयत्नाद्-

आकुण्च्पापानमूलं हुतबहसदृश तंतुवत्सूक्ष्मरूपम् ।

तद्बद्ध्वा हृत्सरोजे तदनु दलणके तालु के ब्रह्मरंध्रे

भित्वाते यांति शून्यं प्रविशति गगने यत्र देवो महेशः ॥७८॥

nābhau saṃyamya pavanagatimadho rodhayaṃsaṃprayatnād-

ākuñcyāpānamūlaṃ hutabahasadṛśa tantuvatsūkṣmarūpam /

tadbaddhvā hṛtsaroje tadanu dalaṇake tāluke brahmaraṃdhre

bhitvāte yānti śūnyaṃ praviśati gagane yatra devo maheśaḥ

//78//

A yogī should concentrate on the navel (i.e. *maṇipura cakra*) and powerfully contract the root of the *apāna* below and force it to move upward and unite it with the mind and *prāna*. Again, in that union he should concentrate on the subtle form of light similar to flaming fire. By doing that, the light reaches *anāhata cakra* after penetrating the *maṇipura cakra*, and when the practice is perfected, the light reaches *brahmarandhra* (the opening at the crown of the head) after penetrating the *anāhata cakra*. Again, at the time of giving up the body (of the yogī) it abandons *brahmarandhra* and enters into the space of void, and there it dissolves into *Deva Mahesa* (literally, the Great God, i.e. *Siva*). -2.78

नाभौ शुभ्रारविंद तदुपरि विमलं मंडलं चण्डरश्मे:
संसारस्यैकरूपां त्रिभुवनजननीं धर्मदात्रीं नराणाम् ।
तस्मिनमध्ये त्रिमार्गे त्रितयतनुधरां छिन्नमस्तां प्रशस्तां
तां वंदे ज्ञानरूपां मरणभयहरां योगिनीज्ञानमुद्राम् ॥७९॥

nābhau śubhrāravindaṃ tadupari vimalaṃ maṇḍalaṃ caṇḍaraśmeḥ

saṃsārasyaikarūpāṃ tribhuvanajananīṃ dharmadātrīṃ narāṇām /

tasminamadhye trimārge tritayatanudharāṃ chinnamastāṃ praśastāṃ

tāṃ vande jñānarūpāṃ maraṇabhayaharāṃ yoginījñānamudrām //79//

The pure rays from the disk of sun are above the bright lotus at the navel where I revere the Goddess (*Kuṇḍalini*) who is in one universal form, is the mother of the three worlds, the bestower of the truth to human beings, and has three qualities; who branches into three paths and three bodily forms, and is praised as *Chinnamastā* (the beheaded form of the Goddess) who is in the form of wisdom, the destroyer of the fear of death, and is the Supreme *Yoginī* in the form of wisdom. - 2.79

Supremacy of Dhyāna Yoga

अश्वमेधसहस्राणि वाजपेयशतानि च ।
एकस्य ध्यानयोगस्य तुलां नार्हन्ति षोडशीम् ॥८०॥

aśvamedhasahasrāṇi vājapeyaśatāni ca /

ekasya dhyānayogasya tulāṃ nārhanti ṣoḍaśīm //80//

A thousand *Aśvamedha Yajñas* (literally, a horse sacrifice which required one full year to complete, performed to fulfill one's wishes) and a hundred *Vājapeya Yajñas* (a special sacrifice which used to be performed by the kings to gain sovereign power) are not equivalent to one sixteenth of *dhyānayoga* (the yoga of meditation, literally, union through meditation). -2.80

Description of Samādhi

उपाधिश्च तथा तत्त्वं द्वयमेतदुदाहृतम् ।

उपाधिः प्रोच्यते वर्णस्तत्त्वमात्माभिधीयते ॥८१॥

upādhiśca tathā tattvaṃ dvayametadudāhṛtam /

upādhiḥ procyate varṇastatvamātmābhidhīyate //81//

Upādhi (superimposition) and *Tattva* (literally, essence, real nature, the Truth, i.e. Supreme Spirit) are the two topics described here. *Upādhi* (superimposition) is said to be *varṇa* (literally, coloring, i.e. covering) and *Tattva* (the reality) is called *Ātmā* (the Self). -2.81

उपाधेरन्यथा ज्ञानतत्त्वसंस्थितिरन्यथा ।

समस्तोपाधिविध्वंसी सदाभ्यासेन जायते ॥८२॥

upādheranyathā jñānatatvasaṃsthitiranyathā /

samastopādhividhvaṃsī sadābhyāsena jāyate //82//

Upādhi (superimposition) creates misunderstanding. In contrast, when wisdom is acquired, then the reality (the Self) is known. Through constant practice and right understanding, all types of superimpositions are destroyed. -2.82

Distinction between Dhyāna and Samādhi

शब्दादीनां च तंमात्रं यावत्कर्णादिषु स्थितम् ।

तावदेवं स्मृतं ध्यानं समाधिः स्यादतः परम् ॥८३॥

śabdādīnāṃ ca tanmātraṃ yāvatkarṇādiṣu sthitam /

tāvadevaṃ smṛtaṃ dhyānaṃ samādhiḥ syādataḥ param //83//

So long as the subject matters of the senses and their objects present in the mind through their respective senses (i.e. the sounds in ears, etc.) it is considered *smṛti dhyāna* (recollective state of meditation). Ultimately, one attains the supreme state of *samādhi* (superconscious state) when the mind and its waves generated through the senses are totally dissolved into *Ātmā* (the Self). -2.83

धारण पञ्चनाडीभिर्ध्यानं च षष्टिनाडीभिः ।

दिनद्वादशकेन स्यात्समाधिः प्राणसंयमात् ॥८४॥

dhāraṇā pañcanāḍībhirdhyānaṃ ca ṣaṣṭināḍībhiḥ /

dinadvādaśakena syātsamādhiḥ prāṇasaṃyamāt //84//

Dhāraṇā (concentration) is achieved in *pañcanāḍī* (two hours), *dhyāna* (meditation) is attained in *ṣaṣṭināḍī* (twenty-four hours) and *samādhi* (superconscious state of mind) is accomplished in *dinadvādaśa* (twelve days) through the control of the *prāna* (life force). -2.84

Instances Relating to Samādhi

यत्सर्वं द्वंद्वयोरैक्यं जीवात्मपरमात्मनोः ।

समस्तनष्टसंकल्पः समाधि साभिधीयते ॥८५॥

yatsarvam dvandvayoraikyaṃ jīvātmaparamātmanoḥ /

samastanaṣṭasaṃkalpaḥ samādhi so 'bhidhīyate //85//

When all *dvandas* (pairs of opposites i.e. heat and cold, gain and loss, etc.) become alike, and *Jīvatma* and *Paramātma* become united together and all types of *saṅkalpa* (ideations) are totally eliminated, it is known as *samādhi* (superconscious state of mind). -2.85

अंबुसैंधवयोरैक्यं यथा भवति योगतः ।

तथात्ममनसोरैक्यं समाधिः सोऽभिधीयते ॥८६॥

aṃbusaimdhavayoraikyaṃ yathā bhavati yogataḥ /

tathātmamanasoraikyaṃ samādhiḥ so'bhidhīyate //86//

It is just like when salt is added to water, and they become one. Similarly, the union of the mind with the Self is described as *samādhi* (superconscious state). -2.86

यदा संक्षीयते प्राणो मानसं च प्रलीयते ।

यदा समरसत्वं च समाधि सोऽभिधीयते ॥८७॥

yadā saṅkṣīyate prāṇo mānasaṃ ca pralīyate /

yadā samarasatvaṃ ca samādhi so'bhidhīyate //87//

It is described as *samādhi* (superconscious state) when *prāna* is diminished totally, mind is absorbed completely, and *samarasatva* (a harmonious state) is established between the *Jīvātmā* (the Embodied Self) and *Paramātmā* (the Supreme Self). -2.87

Absence of Objective World in Samādhi

न गंधं न रसं रूपं न च स्पर्शं न निःस्वनम् ।

नात्मानं न परस्वं च योगी युक्तः समधिना ॥८८॥

na gaṃdhaṃ na rasaṃ rūpaṃ na ca sparśaṃ na niḥsvanam /

nātmānaṃ na parasvaṃ ca yogī yuktaḥ samadhinā //88//

The yogī who is dissolved in *samādhi* (superconscious state) does not have knowledge of sense-objects i.e. smell, taste, form, touch and sound, or of himself or another. -2.88

अभेद्यः सर्वशस्त्राणाग्वध्यः सर्वदेहिनाम् ।

अग्राह्यो मंत्रयंत्राणां योगी युक्तः समाधिना ॥८९॥

abhedyaḥ sarvaśastrāṇāmavadhyaḥ sarvadehinām /

agrāhyo mantrayantrāṇāṃ yogī yuktaḥ samādhinā //89//

The yogī, who is dissolved in *samādhi* (superconscious state), cannot be penetrated by any type of weapon, harmed by any being or affected by the spell of any mantra and use of any *yantra*. -2.89

बाध्यते न स कालेन लिप्यते न स कर्मणा ।

साध्यते न च केनापि योगीः युक्तः समाधिना ॥९०॥

bādhyate na sa kālena lipyate na sa karmaṇā /

sādhyate na ca kenāpi yogīḥ yuktaḥ samādhinā //90//

The yogī, who is dissolved in *samādhi* (superconscious state), cannot be bound by time, stained by action or controlled by anyone. -2.90

युक्ताहारविहारस्य युक्तचेष्टस्य कर्मसु ।

युक्तस्वप्रावबोधस्य योगो भवति दुखहा ॥९१॥

yuktāhāravihārasya yuktaceṣṭasya karmasu /

yuktasvapnāvabodhasya yogo bhavati dukhahā //91//

Yoga becomes the destroyer of suffering to him who is moderate in eating and recreation, in his effort for work, and in sleep and wakefullness. -2.91

निराद्यन्तं निरालम्बं निष्प्रपञ्चं निरामयम् ।

निराश्रयं निराकारं तत्वं जानति योगवित् ॥९२॥

nirādyantaṃ nirālambaṃ niṣprapañcaṃ nirāmayam /

nirāśrayaṃ nirākāraṃ tatvaṃ jānati yogavit //92//

The expert yogī knows that the Reality is without beginning and end, without support, free from illusion and fault, without (need of any) shelter or protection and formless. -2.92

निर्मलं निश्चलं नित्यं निष्क्रियं निर्गुणं महत् ।

व्योमाविज्ञानमानन्दं ब्रह्मं ब्रह्मविदो विदुः ॥९३॥

nirmalam niścalam nityam niṣkriyam nirguṇam mahat /

vyomāvijñānamānandam brahmam brahmavido viduḥ //93//

The *Brahma* (i.e. the Absolute) is known as pure, immovable, inactive, attributeless, ultimate, space, beyond the knowledge (of the mind and intellect) and blissful according to the experts of the Absolute. -2.93

हेतुदृष्टान्तनिर्मुक्तं मनोबुद्ध्योरगोचरम् ।

व्योम विज्ञानमानन्दं तत्वं तत्वविदो विदुः ॥९४॥

hetudṛṣṭāntanirmuktam manobuddhyoragocaram /

vyoma vijñānamānandam tatvam tatvavido viduḥ //94//

The Reality is outside of *hetu* and *dṛṣṭānta* (logical reason and evidence), not perceptible by *mana* and *buddhi* (the mind and intellect). It is space, consciousness and bliss according to the experts of *Tattva* (Reality). -2.94

Attainment of Beatific State by Yoga

निरातङ्के निरालम्बे निराधारे निरामये ।

योगी योगविधानेन परे ब्रह्मणि लीयते ॥९५॥

nirātaṅke nirālambe nirādhāre nirāmaye /

yogī yogavidhānena pare brahmaṇi līyate //95//

The yogī, through the prescribed methods of yoga, is dissolved into the *Brahman* (Supreme Absolute), which is free from fear, without support, without foundation and faultless. -2.95

यथा घृते घृतं क्षिप्तं घृतमेव हि जायते ।

क्षीरं क्षीरे तथा योगी तत्त्वमेव हि जायते ॥९६॥

yathā ghṛte ghṛtaṃ kṣiptaṃ ghṛtameva hi jāyate /

kṣīraṃ kṣīre tathā yogī tattvameva hi jāyate //96//

Just like ghee poured into ghee disappears and only ghee remains, milk poured into milk disappears and only milk remains, so the yogī becomes one with the Reality. -2.96

दुग्धे क्षीरं धृते सर्पिरग्नौ वह्निरिवार्पितः ।

तन्मयत्वं व्रजत्येवं योगी लीनः परे पदे ॥९७॥

dugdhe kṣīraṃ dhṛte sarpiragnau vahnirivārpitaḥ /

tanmayatvaṃ vrajatyevaṃ yogī līnaḥ pare pade //97//

The form of a yogī, dissolved into *Parama Pada* (the Highest State), becomes identical to *Parabrahma* (the Supreme Reality) just like the milk in milk, the ghee in ghee and the fire into fire. -2.97

भवभयहरं नृणां मुक्तिसोपानसंज्ञकम् ।

गुह्याद् गुह्यतर गुह्यं गोरक्षेण प्रकाशितम् ॥९८॥

bhavabhayaharaṃ nṛṇāṃ muktisopānasaṃjñakam /

guhyād guhyatara guhyaṃ gorakṣeṇa prakāśitam //98//

The mystery (*guhya*) disclosed by *Gorakṣa*, is the highest mystery which is known as the ladder to liberation for men that destroys the fear of the rounds of death and birth). -2.98

गोरक्षसंहितामेतां योगभूतां जनः पठेत् ।

सर्वपापविनिर्मुक्तो योगसिद्धिं लभेद् ध्रुवम् ॥९९॥

gorakṣasaṃhitāmetāṃ yogabhūtāṃ janaḥ paṭhet /

sarvapāpavinirmukto yogasiddhiṃ labhed dhruvam //99//

One devoted to yoga should study this *Gorakṣa Saṃhitā* (the Compilation of *Gorakṣa*) made with the essence of yoga. They will certainly attain freedom from all sins and achieve *yogasiddhi* (perfection in yoga). -2.99

योगशास्त्रं पठेन्नित्यं किमान्यैः शास्त्रविस्तरैः ।

यत्स्वयं आदिनाथस्य निर्गतं वदनाम्बुजात् ॥१००॥

yogaśāstraṃ paṭhennityaṃ kimāanyaiḥ śāstravistaraiḥ /

yatsvayaṃ ādināthasya nirgataṃ vadanāmbujāt //100//

One should regularly study this *Yogaśāstra* (the sacred Yoga Scripture), which has come out of the lotus mouth of *Ādinātha* (i.e. Lord *Śiva*) himself. There is no need/use for extensive studies of other scriptures. -2.100

Fulfillment of Ultimate Goal by Yoga Śāstra

स्नातं तेन समस्ततीर्थसलिलं दत्ता द्विजेभ्यो धरा

यज्ञानां च हुतं सहस्रमयुतं दे वाश्च सम्पूजिताः ।

स्वाद्वन्नेन सुतर्पिताश्च पितरः स्वर्ग च नीताः पुन

यस्य ब्रह्मविचारणे क्षणमपि प्राप्नोति धैर्यं मनः ॥१०१॥

snātaṃ tena samastatīrthasalilaṃ dattā dvijebhyo dharā

yajñānāṃ ca hutaṃ sahasramayutaṃ devāśca sampūjitāḥ /

svādvannena sutarpitāśca pitaraḥ svarga ca nītāḥ puna

yasya brahmavicāraṇe kṣaṇamapi prāpnoti dhairyaṃ manaḥ //101//

Suppose one who studied this *Yogaśāstra* completed the holy baths of all the religious places, donated the earth to priests, offered oblations to thousands of sacrifices, worshiped all the Gods and deities, and helped his ancestors attain heavenly abode again having offered libations of water to them. This is because all the above-mentioned results are instantly attained through the study of it (the *Yogaśāstra*) with a calm mind. -2.101

इति श्रीगोरक्षयोगशास्त्रे उत्तरशतकम् ॥

iti śrīgorakṣayogaśāstre uttaraśatakam //

Thus ends the Second Part of *Gorakṣa Yogaśāstra.*